BLOOD TRANSFUSION

A Physician's Handbook
Seventh Edition

American Association of Blood Banks
2002

Editor

Darrell J. Triulzi, MD

Contributing Editors

Agnes Aysola, MD
Robertson Davenport, MD
Jerome Gottschall, MD
Karen King, MD
Ellen Klapper, MD
Edward L. Snyder, MD

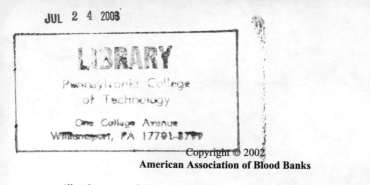
Copyright © 2002
American Association of Blood Banks

American Association of Blood Banks
8101 Glenbrook Road
Bethesda, Maryland 20814

ISBN NO. 1-56395-161-4
Printed in the United States of America
2002

Contents

Preface

The *Blood Transfusion Therapy: A Physician's Handbook* has been revised to help keep medical and paramedical professionals aware of recent developments in transfusion medicine. The seventh edition of the *BTT Handbook* is in compliance with the 21st edition of the AABB *Standards for Blood Banks and Transfusion Services*. The entire *BTT Handbook* has been carefully reviewed and rewritten to reflect state-of-the-art transfusion medicine practices.

A new chapter on Therapeutic Apheresis has been added to emphasize the important role of this therapy in treating a wide variety of illnesses. The chapter provides a practical review of the indications, technical considerations and complications of apheresis therapy. The Blood Components chapter describes the content and indications for each of the major blood components, including new sections on oxygen therapeutics and the emerging technologies for pathogen reduction of blood components. The Plasma Derivatives chapter includes new information on recombinant Factor VII and activated Protein C preparations.

The Transfusion Practices chapter reflects current thinking about a wide variety of transfusion issues, including alternatives to allogeneic transfusion, platelet refractoriness, pediatric transfusion therapy, and transfusion support in solid organ transplantation. The revised Hemostatic Disorders chapter has been updated to relay current knowledge of the role of recently described risk factors for thrombosis including mutations in Factor V and II genes and elevated Factor VIII levels. The chapter on Adverse Effects of Blood Transfusion has been updated with important new topics, including drug-induced hemolysis, sickle cell hemolytic reactions, and posttransfusion purpura. The section on transfusion-transmitted diseases has been expanded to incorporate new information on known viruses and recognize the emerging importance of new pathogens such as prions and parasites (eg, Chagas' disease).

Finally, the chapter on Hematopoietic Progenitor Cells has been revised to reflect the recent advances in this increasingly important area of transfusion medicine, including discussions of new growth factors, cord blood transplantation, and donor leuko-cyte infusions. Readers will also find a new table providing guidance on the selection of blood components in ABO-mismatched hematopoietic cell transplantation.

As in the past, the *BTT Handbook* is intended to serve as a convenient reference for issues relating to transfusion medicine; therefore, the format remains the same concise discussions with references provided for further information. While an attempt has been made to provide some background information, the need for brevity in such a book precludes the presentation of material in exhaustive detail. The reference lists that conclude each chapter serve as good starting points for readers seeking additional details. Although the *BTT Handbook* necessarily reflects the views of the authors, we have attempted to identify controversial topics clearly and to present an unbiased view of current practices. The editors gratefully acknowledge the support of the many people who have made this revised edition possible, especially our AABB staff liaison, Janet McGrath.

BLOOD COMPONENTS

Concept of Blood Component Therapy

Blood component therapy refers to the transfusion of the specific part of blood that the patient needs, as opposed to the routine transfusion of Whole Blood. Because one donated unit can benefit several patients, this procedure not only conserves blood resources, but also provides the optimal method of transfusing patients who require large amounts of a specific blood component. A unit of Whole Blood can be processed through a series of centrifugation steps into units of Red Blood Cells (RBCs), Platelets, and Fresh Frozen Plasma or Cryoprecipitated AHF (see Table 1). The plasma can also be used to manufacture several blood derivatives (eg, concentrates of coagulation factors, immune globulin, and plasma volume expanders), which are then treated to reduce or eliminate the risk of virus transmission. Apheresis technology can also be used to collect red cells, plasma, and/or platelets.[1] Enough platelets for a single transfusion can be obtained by processing blood from a single donor by apheresis, thereby limiting the risk of disease transmission. Thus, the availability of blood components and derivatives permits patients to receive specific hemotherapy that is more effective and usually safer than the use of Whole Blood.

During manufacture, the entire blood bag and any integrally attached satellite bags and needles are sterilized. Because the entire blood collection system is sterile, disposable, and never reused, it is impossible for a donor to contract any disease by donating blood. The blood collection set (including some apheresis systems) is considered a closed system, being open only at the tip of the needle used for donor phlebotomy. When the administra-

Table 1. Blood Components and Plasma Derivatives

Component/ Product	Composition	Volume	Indications
Whole Blood	RBCs (approx. Hct 40%); plasma; WBCs; platelets	500 mL	Increase both red cell mass and plasma volume (WBCs and platelets not functional; plasma deficient in labile clotting Factors V and VIII)
Red Blood Cells	RBC (approx. Hct 75%); reduced plasma, WBCs, and platelets	250 mL	Increase red cell mass in symptomatic anemia (WBCs and platelets not functional)
Red Blood Cells, Adenine-Saline Added	RBC (approx. Hct 60%); reduced plasma, WBCs, and platelets; 100 mL of additive solution	330 mL	Increase red cell mass in symptomatic anemia (WBCs and platelets not functional)
RBCs Leukocytes Reduced (prepared by filtration)	>85% original volume of RBC; $<5 \times 10^6$ WBC; few platelets; minimal plasma	225 mL	Increase red cell mass; $<5 \times 10^6$ WBCs to decrease the likelihood of febrile reactions, immunization to leukocytes (HLA antigens) or CMV transmission
RBCs Washed	RBCs (approx. Hct 75%); $<5 \times 10^8$ WBCs; no plasma	180 mL	Increase red cell mass; reduce risk of allergic reactions to plasma proteins

RBCs Frozen; RBCs Deglycerolized	RBC (approx. Hct 75%); $<5 \times 10^8$ WBCs; no platelets; no plasma	180 mL	Increase red cell mass; minimize febrile or allergic transfusion reactions; use for prolonged RBC blood storage
Granulocytes Pheresis	Granulocytes ($>1.0 \times 10^{10}$ PMN/unit); lymphocytes; platelets ($>2.0 \times 10^{11}$/unit); some RBCs	220 mL	Provide granulocytes for selected patients with sepsis and severe neutropenia (<500 PMN/μL)
Platelets	Platelets ($>5.5 \times 10^{10}$/unit); RBC; WBCs; plasma	50 mL	Bleeding due to thrombocytopenia or thrombocytopathy
Platelets Pheresis	Platelets ($>3 \times 10^{11}$/unit); RBCs; WBCs; plasma	300 mL	Same as Platelets; sometimes HLA matched
Platelets Leukocytes Reduced	Platelets (as above); $<5 \times 10^6$ WBCs per final dose of pooled Platelets	300 mL	Same as Platelets; $<5 \times 10^6$ WBCs to decrease the likelihood of febrile reactions, alloimmunization to leukocytes (HLA antigens), or CMV transmission
FFP; Donor Retested Plasma; Thawed Plasma	FFP, Donor Retested Plasma; all coagulation factors; Thawed Plasma has reduced Factors V and VIII	220 mL	Treatment of some coagulation disorders

(Continued)

3

Table 1. Blood Components and Plasma Derivatives (Continued)

Component/Product	Composition	Volume	Indications
Cryoprecipitated AHF	Fibrinogen; Factors VIII and XIII; von Willebrand factor	15 mL	Deficiency of fibrinogen; Factor XIII; second choice in treatment of Hemophilia A, von Willebrand disease; topical fibrin sealant
Factor VIII (concentrates; recombinant human Factor VIII)	Factor VIII; trace amount of other plasma proteins (products vary in purity)	25 mL	Hemophilia A (Factor VIII deficiency); von Willebrand disease (off-label use for selected products only)
Factor IX (concentrates, recombinant human Factor IX)	Factor IX; trace amount of other plasma proteins (products vary in purity)	25 mL	Hemophilia B (Factor IX deficiency)
Albumin/PPF	Albumin, some α-, β-globulins	(5%); (25%)	Volume expansion

Component	Description	Volume	Indications
Immune Globulin	IgG antibodies; preparations for IV and/or IM use	Varies	Treatment of hypo- or agammaglobulinemia; disease prophylaxis; autoimmune thrombocytopenia (IV only)
Rh Immune Globulin	IgG anti-D; preparations for IV and/or IM use	1 mL	Prevention of hemolytic disease of the newborn due to D antigen; treatment of autoimmune thrombocytopenia
Antithrombin	Antithrombin; trace amount of other plasma proteins	10 mL	Treatment of antithrombin deficiency
Activated Protein C (recombinant)	Activated Protein C		Severe sepsis
Factor VIIa (recombinant)	Factor VIIa	2.2 mL (1.2 mg)/8.5 mL (4.8 mg)	Bleeding episodes for hemophilia A or B with inhibitors

RBCs = red blood cells; Hct = hematocrit; WBCs = white blood cells; CMV = cytomegalovirus; PMN = polymorphonuclear leukocytes; FFP = fresh frozen plasma; PPF = plasma protein fraction; IV = intravenous; IM = intramuscular

tion ports of a blood bag have been opened, however, the unit is considered an open system and should be transfused within 4 hours to avoid possible bacterial contamination. To prepare components that have the maximum permitted shelf life, integral satellite bags must be used to ensure maintenance of the closed system. Alternatively, sterile connection devices are available; these devices permit sterile attachment of separate plastic bags.

Whole Blood

Description of Component

A unit of Whole Blood contains approximately 500 mL of blood and 70 mL of anticoagulant-preservative. The hematocrit of a typical unit is 36% to 44%. Whole Blood is stored in a monitored refrigerator at 1 to 6 C. The shelf life of Whole Blood is dictated by the recovery rate of the transfused red cells 24 hours after infusion; this value must average $\geq$ 75%. For this reason, the shelf life of Whole Blood depends on the preservative used in the blood collection bag [the shelf life of blood in citrate-phosphate-dextrose (CPD) is 21 days; that blood in CPD-adenine (CPDA-1) is 35 days]. See Table 2.

The level of 2,3-diphosphoglycerate (2,3-DPG), an intracytoplasmic molecule that facilitates the release of oxygen from hemoglobin, decreases during storage and is regenerated after infusion of the blood.[2] Whole Blood stored longer than 24 hours contains few viable platelets or granulocytes. In addition, levels of Factor V and Factor VIII decrease with storage. Levels of stable clotting factors, however, are well-maintained in units of Whole Blood during storage.

Indications

Whole Blood provides both oxygen-carrying capacity and blood volume expansion. The primary indication is for treating patients

Table 2. Characteristics of Whole Blood Stored for 35 Days in CPDA-1 (N=10)*

	Storage Time (Days)				
	0	7	14	21	35
Plasma dextrose (mg/dL)	432.0	374.0	357.0	324.0	282.0
Plasma sodium (mEq/L)	169.0	162.0	159.0	157.0	153.0
Plasma potassium (mEq/L)	3.3	12.3	17.6	21.7	17.2
Plasma chloride (mEq/L)	84.0	81.0	79.0	77.0	79.0
Plasma bicarbonate (mEq/L)	12.0	17.0	12.5	12.2	8.0
Whole-blood pH	7.16	6.94	6.93	6.87	6.73
Whole-blood lactate (mg/dL)	19.0	62.0	91.0	130.0	202.0
Plasma LDH (units)	296.0	1002.0	1222.0	1457.0	1816.0
Whole-blood ammonia (mg/dL)	82.0	280.0	423.0	521.0	703.0
Plasma hemoglobin (mg/dL)	0.5	13.1	24.7	24.7	45.6
WBC (103/mL)	7.2	4.0	3.0	2.8	2.4
Hematocrit (%)	35.0	36.0	35.0	36.0	36.0
RBC hemoglobin (g/dL)	12.0	12.0	12.0	12.0	12.0
RBC (106/mL)	4.0	4.0	3.9	3.9	3.9
Red blood cell 2,3-DPG (mmol/gHb)[†]	13.2	—	—	—	0.7
Red blood cell ATP (mmol/gHb)	4.18	—	—	—	2.40

*Latham JT, Bove JR, Weirich FL. Chemical and hematologic changes in stored CPDA-1 blood. Transfusion 1982;22:158-9.
[†]Moore GL, Peck CC, Sohmer PR, Zuck TF. Some properties of blood stored in anticoagulant CPDA-1 solution. Transfusion 1981;21:135-7.

who are actively bleeding and who have sustained a loss of greater than 25% of their total blood volume. Such patients may develop hemorrhagic shock. In some regions, blood centers maintain inventories of Whole Blood for use in massively bleeding patients (those transfused one blood volume, or more than 10 units of RBCs in less than 24 hours). This use may limit donor exposures if RBCs and Fresh Frozen Plasma (FFP) would otherwise be given (see Urgent and Massive Transfusion). Unless a patient needs volume replacement in addition to oxygen-carrying capacity, the use of Whole Blood may result in fluid overload, especially if rapid infusion is attempted. If platelets or granulocytes are required, the appropriate cellular components should be used. Plasma should be given to replace needed labile clotting factors. Whole Blood less than 7 days old may be beneficial for neonatal exchange transfusions to prevent hyperkalemia. There is limited justification for use of "fresh" Whole Blood (ie, blood collected within the previous 48 hours) specifically for infants undergoing certain complex cardiac surgical procedures.

Contraindications and Precautions

Whole Blood should not be given to patients with chronic anemia who are normovolemic and require only an increase in red cell mass; RBCs should be used for such patients to decrease the risk of blood volume overload. See Chapter 5: Adverse Effects of Transfusion.

Dose and Administration

In an adult, one unit of Whole Blood will increase the hemoglobin level by about 1 g/dL or the hematocrit by about 3% to 4%. In pediatric patients, a Whole Blood transfusion of 8 mL/kg will result in an increase in hemoglobin of approximately 1 g/dL. Whole Blood must be administered through a blood administration set containing a 150- to 280-micron filter. The rate of infusion depends on the clinical condition of the patient, but each unit or aliquot should be infused within 4 hours.

Red Blood Cells

Description of Component

RBCs are prepared from Whole Blood by the removal of 200 to 250 mL of plasma or they may be obtained by apheresis collection. They are stored at 1 to 6 C in one of several anticoagulant-preservative solutions. These solutions contain varying amounts and/or types of preservative agents (eg, buffer, dextrose, adenine, and mannitol). The resultant RBC components have different hematocrits and shelf lives. RBCs stored in additive solutions (AS) have hematocrits of 52% to 60% and a shelf life of 42 days, whereas RBCs stored in CPDA-1 have hematocrits of 70% to 80% and can be stored for 35 days.[2-4] RBCs stored in CPD have hematocrits similar to those of RBCs stored in CPDA-1, but with a shelf life of 21 days. RBCs are not a source of functional platelets or granulocytes. RBCs and Whole Blood have the same oxygen-carrying capacity because they contain the same number of red cells.

Indications

RBCs are indicated for treatment of anemia in normovolemic patients who require an increase in oxygen-carrying capacity and red cell mass. The transfusion requirements of each patient should be based on clinical status rather than on any predetermined hematocrit or hemoglobin value.[5] RBCs, rather than Whole Blood, are advantageous for patients who do not require or cannot tolerate excessive volume expansion, such as anemic patients with cardiac failure.

Contraindications and Precautions

Risks associated with RBC infusion are the same as those encountered with Whole Blood. See Chapter 5: Adverse Effects of Blood Transfusion.

Dose and Administration

In an adult with an average blood volume, one unit of RBCs will increase the hemoglobin level by about 1 g/dL or the hematocrit by about 3%. In a pediatric patient an RBC transfusion of 8-10 mL/kg will raise the hemoglobin level about 2 g/dL or the hematocrit by about 6%. RBCs must be transfused through use of a blood administration filter (150 to 280 microns). The higher hematocrit of CPD or CPDA-1 RBCs results in increased viscosity, which may slow the transfusion rate. To decrease viscosity, 50-100 mL of isotonic sodium chloride (0.9% USP) may be used to dilute the RBCs in CPD or CPDA-1, but this practice must be balanced against the risk of hypervolemia. The lower hematocrit of the RBCs in AS units permits more rapid infusion rates. For patients at risk for circulatory overload and for pediatric patients, concern over the additional volume resulting from the 100 mL of additive solution may warrant concentrating the component by centrifugation or sedimentation. Other than isotonic saline, no solutions or medications should be added to RBCs (see Administration of Blood in Chapter 3).

Red Blood Cells Leukocytes Reduced

Description of Component

Units of RBCs contain 1 to 3×10^9 leukocytes.[6,7] AABB *Standards for Blood Banks and Transfusion Services*[1] specifies that leukocyte-reduced RBCs must contain $<5 \times 10^6$ leukocytes/unit while retaining 85% of the original red cells. The standard 170-micron blood filter does not remove leukocytes, but third-generation leukocyte reduction filters, when properly employed, enable this requirement to be met. Leukocyte reduction may be performed at the time of transfusion by passing the blood through one of several commercially available third-generation bedside blood filters, which usually leaves $<5 \times 10^6$ leukocytes in the transfused blood.[8] The success of this method depends on the duration of unit storage, the initial leukocyte content of the unit, and the proper use of the filter.

Leukocyte reduction is best achieved by filtration of the unit in the blood center shortly after blood collection (prestorage filtration), or in the transfusion service laboratory before blood issue (laboratory filtration). These methods have several potential advantages when compared with bedside filtration of RBCs. Laboratory filtration is generally more effective than bedside filtration, consistently leaving $<10^6$ leukocytes/unit. It can provide an immediately available inventory of Red Blood Cells Leukocytes Reduced with a normal shelf life, and it permits quality control of residual leukocyte content.[9,10] Greater numbers of bedside-filtered units fail to meet current leukocyte reduction standards (commonly due to high donor leukocyte counts or to improper use). Bedside filtration may be unacceptable for surgical patients because of the slow rate of blood passage through the filter. Prestorage leukocyte reduction results in lower levels of cytokine generation in blood bags during storage and may result in a lower risk of febrile nonhemolytic transfusion reactions.[11-13]

Indications

Red Blood Cells Leukocytes Reduced are indicated for patients who have had repeated febrile reactions in association with the transfusion of RBCs or Platelets, and as prophylaxis against alloimmunization in selected patients in whom intensive or long-term hemotherapy is anticipated.[10] Patients who have received frequent transfusions and women who have had multiple pregnancies may become alloimmunized to leukocyte antigens. Alloimmunization can be manifested as febrile transfusion reactions and/or as refractoriness to platelet transfusion (see Platelets). Studies indicate that leukocytes are responsible for the development of alloimmunization to HLA antigens[14] and that antibodies to leukocyte antigens are responsible for many recurrent febrile transfusion reactions, as well as the development of transfusion-related acute lung injury (see Chapter 5: Adverse Effects of Blood Transfusion).[15] Patients who have febrile nonhemolytic transfusion reactions should receive leukocyte-reduced blood components. The use of bedside filtration methods employing third-generation filters is successful in preventing recurrent febrile nonhemolytic reactions caused by alloimmunization in most patients.[7,10] For patients who continue to experience recurrent febrile reactions, prestorage leukocyte reduction or laboratory filtration may be effective.

Studies suggest that the routine prophylactic use of filtered leukocyte-reduced blood components diminishes the likelihood of primary alloimmunization to leukocyte antigens.[10,16] Patients who have a high likelihood of becoming alloimmunized (eg, patients with chronic transfusion requirements) may be considered candidates for the prophylactic use of leukocyte-reduced blood components.[10,16] A decision to use leukocyte-reduced red cells prophylactically in an effort to prevent alloimmunization should optimally be made before the first blood transfusion. The decision implies a commitment to use leukocyte-reduced Platelets as well as RBCs (see Platelets Leukocytes Reduced).

Certain immunosuppressed, cytomegalovirus (CMV)-seronegative patients such as allogeneic hematopoietic progenitor cell transplant recipients are susceptible to severe transfusiontransmitted CMV disease.[17] Clinical studies of such patients indicate that leukocyte-reduced blood components prepared by third-generation filters are as effective in preventing transmission of CMV infection as are blood components obtained from CMV-seronegative donors.[18-20]

Transfusion of cellular blood components is associated with changes in host immune function. This property was once employed to prolong the survival of renal allografts, but has been supplanted by improved immunosuppressive drug therapy. Most, but not all, prospective randomized studies have shown that the use of leukocyte-reduced blood reduces the incidence of wound infection in selected surgical patients. However, the mechanism of this effect is unclear and the use of leukocyte reduction filters for this purpose is controversial.[21,22]

Recent recommendations to require leukocyte reduction of all cellular blood components are controversial. Decisions about selective leukocyte reduction should be based on several factors, including therapeutic goals and method of leukocyte reduction. Consultation with the transfusion service physician is recommended.

Contraindications and Precautions

Patients who receive Red Blood Cells Leukocytes Reduced are subject to the same volume-related hazards as those who receive RBCs. Red Blood Cells Leukocytes Reduced may contain 5% to 10% fewer red cells resulting from loss in the filters. This component is not indicated to prevent posttransfusion graft-vs-host disease (GVHD) because cases of GVHD have been reported after its use. Irradiated blood should be used to prevent posttransfusion GVHD. Hypotension has been reported with the use of some bedside filters.

Dose and Administration

Administration of RBCs through a third-generation leukocyte reduction filter at the bedside eliminates the need for the standard blood filter. However, units that are leukocyte-reduced by prestorage filtration or laboratory filtration must be transfused through a blood administration filter. Personnel who administer blood through leukocyte reduction filters should be thoroughly familiar with the requirements for their use in order to achieve optimal leukocyte reduction, provide acceptable blood flow rates, and ensure against excessive loss of red cells.

Red Blood Cells Washed

Description of Component

RBCs may be washed with sterile saline using specially designed machines. The washed red cells are suspended in sterile saline, usually at hematocrits of 70% to 80% with a volume of approximately 180 mL. Saline washing removes all but traces of plasma

(98%), reduces the concentration of leukocytes, and removes platelets and cellular debris. Saline washing may be performed at any time during the shelf life of a unit of blood, but because washing is ordinarily performed in an open system, the resultant red cell component can be stored for only 24 hours at 1 to 6 C.

Indications

The predominant indication for RBCs Washed in adults is to prevent recurrent or severe allergic reactions. This component may also be used in neonatal or intrauterine transfusion. In the past, RBCs Washed were often ordered to provide "leukocyte-reduced" RBCs; however, given the limited efficacy of this method compared with that of current filtration methods, the use of RBCs Washed for this purpose alone is not indicated. RBCs Washed may also be used for patients requiring red cell transfusion who are hyperkalemic.

Contraindications and Precautions

RBCs Washed may be stored at 1 to 6 C for no longer than 24 hours following preparation because of the risk of bacterial contamination.[1] Washing is associated with loss of 10% to 20% of the RBCs. Transfusion hazards associated with washed cells are similar to those of RBCs. RBCs Washed are capable of transmitting hepatitis[23] and other infectious diseases. Because they contain sufficient numbers of viable leukocytes, this component will not prevent posttransfusion GVHD.

Dose and Administration

All units must be infused through a blood administration set containing a 150- to 280-micron filter. Because a unit of RBCs Washed provides a smaller red cell mass than does a unit of RBCs, patients who are chronically transfused with RBCs Washed may require additional transfusions to achieve the desired hematocrit.

Red Blood Cells Frozen; Red Blood Cells Deglycerolized

Description of Component

RBCs Frozen are prepared by adding glycerol, a cryoprotective agent, to blood usually less than 6 days old. The unit is then frozen at -65 or -200 C (depending on the concentration of cryoprotective agent) for as long as 10 years. Once thawed, the unit is washed to remove the glycerol by using a series of saline-glucose solutions. The unit is then reconstituted in sterile saline, usually at a hematocrit of 70% to 80%. When prepared in an open system this component may be stored at 1 to 6 C for no longer than 24 hours.[1] When prepared using a closed system the unit may be stored at 1 to 6 C for 14 days.

Indications

This technique is useful for long-term preservation of RBC units of a rare phenotype and autologous RBCs. In the past, frozen and deglycerolized RBCs were used as a source of leukocyte-reduced blood because they contain <10% of the leukocytes usually found in a unit of RBCs; however, leukocyte reduction filters are now preferred for this purpose.

Contraindications and Precautions

RBCs that have been frozen and deglycerolized carry the same risks and hazards as do Washed RBCs. This component is capable of transmitting infectious diseases (eg, hepatitis) and has been shown to contain viable lymphocytes.[24]

Dose and Administration

All units must be given through a blood administration set with a 150- to 280-micron filter. RBCs Deglycerolized provide a smaller red cell mass because of the loss of red cells during processing.

Therefore, patients transfused with these units could require additional transfusions to achieve a desired hematocrit.

Platelets

PLATELETS

Description of Component

Platelets are prepared from individual units of Whole Blood by centrifugation. Units should contain at least 5.5×10^{10} platelets in sufficient plasma (usually 50 to 70 mL) to maintain a pH greater than 6.2 throughout the storage period.[1] Platelets, which may be stored in the blood bank for as long as 5 days at 20 to 24 C with constant gentle agitation, have nearly normal posttransfusion recovery and survival.[25] They are frequently pooled at the time of issue; if pooled, Platelets must be transfused within 4 hours.

Indications

Platelets are indicated for treatment of bleeding caused by thrombocytopenia (platelet counts usually below 50,000/μL) or for patients with functionally abnormal platelets (congenital or acquired).[26,27] They are also indicated during surgery or before certain invasive procedures in patients who have platelet counts of <50,000/μL. Prophylactic transfusion of Platelets may be indicated for patients who have platelet counts below 5000 to 10,000/μL associated with marrow hypoplasia resulting from chemotherapy, tumor invasion, or primary aplasia.[28-30] This range may be higher for patients with complicating clinical factors.[29] There is no evidence that prophylactic transfusion of platelets is beneficial in massive transfusion[31] or in cardiac surgery.[32]

Contraindications and Precautions

Platelet transfusions may not be effective in patients with rapid platelet destruction. These conditions include idiopathic autoimmune thrombocytopenic purpura (ITP), and untreated disseminated intravascular coagulation (DIC). In such patients, platelet transfusion should be used only in the presence of active bleeding and with careful clinical monitoring. Platelet transfusions are relatively contraindicated in patients with thrombotic thrombocytopenic purpura (TTP) and heparin-induced thrombocytopenia (HIT). Patients with thrombocytopenia caused by septicemia or hypersplenism also may fail to benefit from platelet transfusions.

Chills, fever, and allergic reactions may occur. Fever should not be treated with antipyretics containing aspirin (acetylsalicylic acid), because aspirin will inhibit platelet function. Repeated transfusions may lead to alloimmunization to HLA and other antigens, and may result in the development of a "refractory" state manifested by unresponsiveness to platelet transfusion (see Management of Platelet Alloimmunization). Some transfusion reactions appear to be associated with the accumulation of cytokines in stored platelets, suggesting that the reactions might be prevented by using platelets stored fewer than 3 days or by prestorage leukocyte reduction of platelets.[33,34] Because small amounts of red cells may be present in a platelet transfusion, patients who are D-negative generally should receive only platelets from a D-negative donor. If D-positive Platelets must be transfused to D-negative females of childbearing potential or children, prevention of D immunization by the use of Rh Immune Globulin should be considered. Plasma contained in transfused units of ABO-incompatible Platelets may cause a positive direct antiglobulin test (DAT) result and, very rarely, hemolysis in the recipient.[35] Whenever possible, ABO-compatible Platelets should be selected. Rapid infusion may cause circulatory overload and other complications related to increased intravascular volume. The risks of transfusion-transmitted infectious diseases are similar to those associated with RBCs, and because platelets from multiple donors must be pooled to obtain an adequate dose for an adult, those risks are multiplied. Bacterial contamination of Platelets is of special concern because this component is stored at room temperature.[36]

Dose and Administration

The usual dose for a thrombocytopenic bleeding patient is 1 unit of Platelets per 10 kg body weight (typically 5 to 7 units for an adult). One unit of Platelets usually increases the platelet count in a 70-kg adult by 5000/μL. Repeated failure to achieve hemostasis or the expected increment in platelet count may signify the refractory state.[26,37] Immune refractoriness to platelets is most commonly associated with antibodies to HLA antigens and rarely to platelet-specific antigens. Clinical refractoriness to platelets is associated with bleeding, amphotericin, splenomegaly, DIC, fever, sepsis, or hematopoietic progenitor cell transplantation.[38] Refractoriness is often suspected on the basis of repeatedly poor clinical response to platelet transfusion and a poor posttransfusion platelet count increment. The corrected count increment (CCI) may be calculated more accurately as follows:

$$CCI = \frac{(\text{Post-tx plt ct}) - (\text{Pre-tx plt ct}) \times BSA}{(\text{Platelets transfused} \times 10^{11})}$$

where Pre-tx plt ct = pretransfusion platelet count, Post-tx plt ct = posttransfusion platelet count, and BSA = body surface area in square meters. As an estimate, each unit of Platelets contains 6×10^{10} platelets and a unit of Platelet Pheresis contains 3×10^{11} platelets.

A CCI of >7.5 to 10×10^9/L from a sample drawn 10 minutes to 1 hour after transfusion, or a CCI of >4.5 × 10^9/L from a sample drawn 18 to 24 hours after transfusion is considered acceptable (ie, not indicative of refractoriness).[39,40] Patients who repeatedly have poor clinical or 1-hour CCI responses are more likely to be immune refractory to platelet transfusion and pose difficult management problems (see Management of Platelet Alloimmunization). Patients who are refractory because of the emergence of HLA or platelet alloantibodies usually require HLA-matched or crossmatched platelets.[37] Patients who have adequate

1-hour CCI responses, but poor 24-hour CCI recovery, are most likely refractory due to nonimmune causes and may require more frequent or larger doses of platelets.

Platelets must be administered through a blood administration set with a 150- to 280-micron filter. Testing of platelets for red cell compatibility is not necessary unless visual standards indicate that more than 2 mL of red cells are present. Because platelets contain ABO antigens that may diminish their posttransfusion recovery, it may be preferable to give platelets from donors who are ABO compatible with the patient's plasma. Likewise, it is preferable to give donor plasma that is compatible with recipient's red cells if large amounts are given to recipients with small blood volumes.[35] Platelet units may be pooled before administration, or infused individually. Platelets may be volume-reduced to prevent fluid overload or to diminish the transfusion of ABO-incompatible plasma. Platelets should be transfused no longer than 4 hours after pooling. Gamma irradiated platelets must be selected for patients at risk for GVHD.

PLATELETS PHERESIS

Description of Component

Platelets Pheresis are collected from an individual donor during a 1- to 3-hour cytapheresis procedure, and contain at least 3×10^{11} platelets.[1] This number is equal to 5 to 6 units of Platelets. The volume of plasma in the component varies from 200 to 400 mL. The number of leukocytes and red cells varies with the apheresis technique. Platelets Pheresis collected using recently developed technologies may be considered leukocyte-reduced when quality is controlled under current good manufacturing practice regulations.

Indications

Platelets Pheresis that are either HLA-matched or crossmatch-compatible with the recipient are indicated for patients who are unresponsive to random-donor Platelets because of HLA alloimmunization. Non-HLA-matched Platelets Pheresis are also used for patients who are not refractory, in order to limit donor exposures. Physicians treating patients who are refractory to Platelets should consult with the transfusion service director to determine the best therapeutic alternatives (see Management of Platelet Alloimmunization).

Contraindications and Precautions

Adverse effects and hazards are similar to those for Platelets. When compared with pooled Platelets, Platelets Pheresis have been reported to have a lower risk of bacterial contamination.[41] Acute hemolytic transfusion reactions have been reported with transfusion of Platelets Pheresis containing ABO-incompatible plasma.[42]

Dose and Administration

One unit of Platelets Pheresis will usually increase the platelet count of a 70-kg adult by 30,000 to 60,000/μL. Compatibility testing is the same as for Platelets. Preferably, the donors plasma should be ABO compatible with the recipients red cells if they are not group-specific. Administration is similar to that for Platelets.

PLATELETS LEUKOCYTES REDUCED

Description of Component

Platelets contain leukocytes (approximately $0.5\text{-}1 \times 10^8$/unit of Platelets), which are not removed by the standard 170-micron blood filter.[43-45] Platelets Leukocytes Reduced should contain $\leq 8.3 \times 10^5$ leukocytes per unit and, when pooled, a final dose of less than 5×10^6 leukocytes.[1] The number of leukocytes remaining in the component after leukocyte reduction varies with the type of platelet component, the number of units processed, and the type of leukocyte reduction procedure employed. Passage of platelets through third-generation filters (either at the beside or in the laboratory) generally removes 99.9% of leukocytes and less than 10% of the platelets in the platelet component.[44,45] Cytapheresis instruments are reliably capable of reducing the leukocyte content of Platelets Pheresis to $<5 \times 10^6$/unit.[46,47]

Indications

See the earlier discussion of RBCs Leukocytes Reduced. Platelets Leukocytes Reduced are indicated as prophylaxis against HLA alloimmunization in selected patients who are destined to receive long-term hemotherapy.[16,48] The decision to use Platelets Leukocytes Reduced in an effort to prevent alloimmunization should optimally be made before the first blood transfusion. This decision implies a commitment to use RBCs Leukocytes Reduced to ensure that all cellular components are leukocyte reduced. Platelets Leukocytes Reduced are also effective in reducing the risk of transmitting CMV.[18]

Contraindications and Precautions

Although the use of Platelets Leukocytes Reduced may eliminate febrile reactions in patients who are already alloimmunized to HLA antigens, their use will not improve the low platelet recovery rate or short platelet survival time associated with the use of random-donor platelet transfusion in such patients. Obtaining a good platelet increment in such patients nearly always requires the use of HLA-matched or crossmatched platelets.[48] Clinical studies show that various reactions (eg, chills) are associated with transfusion of platelets that have been stored for several days.[33,34,49] Evidence suggests that such reactions may be due to infusion of cytokines, including interleukins (IL-1, IL-6, IL-8), and tumor necrosis factor-alpha (TNF-α), which have been generated by leukocytes during storage.[49-51] There is no evidence to suggest that these reactions can be prevented by bedside filtration; however, clinical data have shown that prestorage leukocyte reduction can reduce the incidence of such reactions.[13] Other hazards are similar to those for Platelets that have not undergone leukocyte reduction.

Dose and Administration

Personnel who prepare Platelets Leukocytes Reduced or administer platelets through leukocyte reduction filters should be thoroughly familiar with the requirements of their use, which vary from one filter to another. Leukocyte reduction filters are manufactured to be component-specific and care must be taken to ensure that an appropriate filter has been selected for use. The use of a leukocyte reduction filter in the administration set when platelets are transfused at the bedside eliminates the need for any other blood administration filter.

PLATELETS PHERESIS LEUKOCYTES REDUCED

Platelets Pheresis Leukocytes Reduced do not appear to have an advantage over pooled Platelets Leukocytes Reduced in reducing the frequency of alloimmunization and refractoriness in patients requiring long-term transfusion support.[16] See Platelets Leukocytes Reduced.

Granulocytes Pheresis

Description of Component

Granulocytes are usually prepared by cytapheresis of a single donor. They may also be prepared as "buffy coat" preparation from single units of fresh blood for neonatal granulocyte transfusion.[52] Each unit contains $\geq 1.0 \times 10^{10}$ granulocytes, and variable amounts of lymphocytes, platelets, and red cells; the unit is then suspended in 200 to 300 mL of plasma. Hydroxyethyl starch (HES, a sedimenting agent), or corticosteroids may be administered to the door to facilitate granulocyte collection. Administration of granulocyte colony-stimulating factor (G-CSF) to healthy donors can significantly increase the collection of granulocytes to 4 to 8×10^{10} granulocytes/bag.[53,54] Healthy donors who receive G-CSF at doses of 5 to 10 µg/kg may experience side effects such as bone pain, myalgia, arthralgia, nausea/vomiting, or headaches, to a mild or moderate degree.[53,55] These symptoms generally require no treatment or can be treated successfully with acetominophen.[55] Fluid retention has been observed in some donors who receive repeated daily doses of corticosteroids and G-CSF. Granulocytes collected from G-CSF-stimulated donors appear to function normally, although they differ phenotypically from granulocytes collected from unstimulated donors with increased expression of adhesion molecules (CD11b, CD18, CD14) and Fcγ receptors (CD32, CD64).[53] Transfusion of G-CSF-moblized granulocyte components results in measurable increases in peripheral blood granulocyte counts of 1000/μL or more, which are sustained above baseline for 1 to 2 days.[56] The presence of platelets in granulocyte concentrates is often beneficial because many neutropenic patients are also thrombocytopenic.[56] Granulocytes should be stored at 20 to 24 C and transfused as soon as possible, but they must be infused within 24 hours of collection.[57]

Indications

The decision to use granulocytes should be made in consultation with the transfusion service physician. The patient typically has neutropenia ($<0.5 \times 10^9$/L), infection (preferably documented) for 24 to 48 hours, lack of responsiveness to appropriate antibiotics or other modes of therapy, marrow showing myeloid hypoplasia, and a reasonable chance for recovery of marrow function. Granulocyte transfusions may also be beneficial for neonatal patients with sepsis.[58] Randomized studies have suggested that granulocyte transfusions of at least 1×10^{10} per transfusion are of benefit in selected neutropenic patients.[59-61] It has been suggested that clinical response to granulocyte transfusion therapy may be limited by the dose of granulocytes administered, and it is possible that the larger doses obtained with G-CSF-stimulated donors may lead to enhanced therapeutic benefit. Randomized clinical studies with G-CSF-enhanced doses of granulocytes are needed to define the clinical indications and efficacy of this therapy.[60]

Contraindications and Precautions

Successful treatment of the infected neutropenic patient includes appropriate antimicrobial therapy, and/or the use of hematopoietic growth factors, in addition to the consideration of the use of granulocyte transfusions. If recovery of marrow function is doubtful, granulocyte transfusions are unlikely to alter the ultimate clinical course of a neutropenic patient. Chills, fever, and allergic reactions may occur, and are minimized by slow infusion rates, diphenhydramine and/or meperidine, steroids, and/or nonaspirin antipyretics. In some patients, severe febrile and pulmonary reactions to Granulocytes Pheresis (eg, when infused in conjuction with amphotericin) may preclude their further use.[62] There is a risk of viral disease transmission, especially CMV; immunization to HLA and red cell antigens may occur as well. In most clinical circumstances, gamma irradiation should be performed to prevent GVHD, because gamma irradiation in doses used to prevent GVHD does not impair the function of granulocytes.

Dose and Administration

Although most blood centers do not perform HLA typing on Granulocytes Pheresis, red cell compatibility testing must be performed because of the large number of red cells present. Patients alloimmunized to HLA are less likely to benefit from random-donor granulocytes.[63] A minimum transfusion of $1\text{-}2 \times 10^{10}$ granulocytes per infusion given in four daily doses have been reported to demonstrate clinical benefit.[63] The kinetics of transfused granulocytes from G-CSF-stimulated donors may allow for every-other-day transfusion.[56] A blood administration set with a 150- to 280-micron filter must be used; the use of leukocyte reduction filters is contraindicated.

Plasma Components

Description of Component

Several plasma alternatives can be used for coagulation factor replacement, including Fresh Frozen Plasma (FFP), Donor Retested Plasma, and Thawed Plasma. The most commonly used plasma component, FFP, is prepared from Whole Blood by separating and freezing the plasma within 8 hours of phlebotomy. FFP and Donor Retested Plasma may also be obtained using apheresis procedures. Apheresis technology allows for the collection of the equivalent of 2 units of plasma during a single donation. Plasma may be stored for as long as 1 year at −18 C or colder. The volume of a typical unit is 200 to 250 mL. Under these conditions, loss of Factors V and VIII, the labile clotting factors, is minimal. One mL of FFP contains approximately one unit of coagulation factor activity. Donor Retested Plasma is FFP that has reduced infectivity for human immunodeficiency virus, types 1 and 2 (HIV-1, HIV-2), hepatitis C virus (HCV), hepatitis B virus (HBV), and human T-cell lymphotropic virus, types I and II (HTLV-I, HTLV-II). Donor Retested Plasma reduces the risk of transmitting these viruses because a unit of FFP is held until the donor comes back to donate a second time at least 112 days later. If testing on the second donation is negative, the first unit can be released because the two negative tests span the "window period" in nearly all donors for each virus. Each unit of Donor Retested Plasma represents a single donor exposure. Thawed Plasma is thawed FFP stored for 4 days beyond the outdate of the FFP. The volume is also 200 to 250 mL. The levels of Factor VIII and Factor V decline during storage, although the latter does not fall below the hemostatic level of 35%.[64] Solvent/detergent-treated plasma, a pooled plasma product that has been treated with a solvent and a detergent to eliminate lipid-enveloped viruses, is used in Europe but is being phased out of use in the United States.[65]

Indications

Plasma is indicated for use in bleeding patients or patients undergoing an invasive procedure with multiple coagulation factor deficiencies (eg, those secondary to liver disease, DIC, and the dilutional coagulopathy resulting from massive blood or volume replacement).[27,66] Plasma transfusion is indicated for the rapid reversal of warfarin effect in a bleeding patient or in the setting of emergency surgery. Thawed Plasma may not be the optimal choice for patients with consumptive coagulopathy because of its reduced content of Factor VIII and V. Because minor prolongations in coagulation tests are not usually associated with excessive bleeding, the prothrombin time (PT) or activated partial thromboplastin time (aPTT) should be indicative of factor levels of 30% or lower or International Normalized Ratios of 1.6 or higher before plasma is used (Table 3).[27,66] Plasma is indicated for patients with congenital factor deficiencies for which there is no coagulation concentrate available, such as deficiencies of Factor V, X, or XI. FFP or Donor Retested Plasma may also be used as primary therapy and as the principal replacement solution in plasmapheresis procedures for the treatment of TTP and adult hemolytic uremic syndrome. The cryoprecipitate-reduced fraction of FFP has been employed in refractory cases of TTP.[67]

Contraindications and Precautions

Plasma should not be used to provide blood volume expansion, because this exposes patients unnecessarily to the risk of transfusion-transmitted diseases. Albumin, plasma protein fraction (PPF), or other colloid or crystalloid solutions that do not transmit infection are safer products to use for blood volume expansion. Similarly, Plasma should not be used as a source of protein for nutritionally deficient patients. In general, FFP and Thawed Plasma have a risk of infectious disease transmission equal to that of Whole Blood. Donor Retested Plasma has a reduced risk of transmitting HIV, HBV, and HCV. Certain viruses (eg, CMV and HTLV-I) do not appear to be transmitted by plasma because they are associated exclusively with leukocytes.[68] Allergic reactions can occur with plasma infusion.[69]

Dose and Administration

The dose of plasma depends on the clinical situation and the underlying disease process. When plasma is given for coagulation factor replacement, the dose is 10 to 20 mL/kg (4 to 6 units in an adult). This dose would be expected to increase the level of coagulation factors by 20% immediately after infusion. Smaller doses may suffice in patients with vitamin K deficiency when one cannot wait for the administered vitamin K to take effect. Posttrans-

Table 3. In-Vitro Properties of Blood Clotting Factors

Factor	Plasma Concentration Required for Hemostasis*	Half-Life of Transfused Factor	Recovery in Blood (as % of Amount Transfused)	Stability in Liquid Plasma and Whole Blood (4 C Storage)
I (fibrinogen)	100-150 mg/dL	3-6 days	50%	Stable
II	40 U/dL (40%)	2-5 days	40-80%	Stable
V	10-25 U/dL (15-25%)	15-36 hours	80%	Unstable[†]
VII	5-20 U/dL (5-10%)	2-7 hours	70-80%	Stable
VIII	10-40 U/dL (10-40%)	8-12 hours	60-80%	Unstable[‡]
IX	10-40%	18-24 hours	40-50%	Stable
X	10-20%	1.5-2 days	50%	Stable
XI	15-30%	3-4 days	90-100%	Stable
XII	—	—	—	Stable
XIII	1-5%	6-10 days	5-100%	Stable
vWF	25-50%	3-5 hours	—	Unstable

*Upper limit usually refers to surgical hemostasis.
[†]50% remains at 14 days.
[‡]25% remains at 24 hours.
Adapted from Colman RW. Hemostasis and thrombosis: Basic principles and clinical practice, 3rd ed. Philadelphia: Lippincott, 1993:958 and Rizza ER. Management of patients with inherited blood coagulation defects. In: Bloom AL, Thomas DP, eds. Haemostasis and thrombosis. London: Churchill Livingstone, 1981:371.

fusion assessment of the patient's coagulation status is important, and monitoring of coagulation function with PT, aPTT, or specific factor assays is critical. As with all blood components, plasma must be given through a filter. Plasma thawed at 30 to 37 C should be transfused as soon as possible, but it must be transfused within 24 hours if it is being used as a source of labile coagulation factors. After thawing, FFP and Donor Retested Plasma should be stored at 1 to 6 C. Compatibility testing is not required, but ABO-compatible plasma must be used.

Cryoprecipitated Antihemophilic Factor (AHF)

Description of Component

Cryoprecipitated AHF is a concentrated source of certain plasma proteins. It is prepared by thawing 1 unit of FFP at 1 to 6 C. After it is thawed, the supernatant plasma is removed, leaving the cold precipitated protein plus 10 to 15 mL of plasma in the bag. This material is then refrozen at −18 C or colder within 1 hour and has a shelf life of 1 year. Cryoprecipitated AHF contains concentrated Factor VIII:C (the procoagulant activity), Factor VIII:vWF (von Willebrand factor), fibrinogen, and Factor XIII. Each bag of Cryoprecipitated AHF contains approximately 80 to 120 units of Factor VIII, at least 150 mg of fibrinogen,[1] and about 20% to 30% of the Factor XIII present in the initial unit. Approximately 40% to 70% of the vWF present in the initial unit of FFP is recovered in the cryoprecipitate. The main source of concentrated fibrinogen is Cryoprecipitated AHF.

Indications

Cryoprecipitated AHF may be indicated for the treatment of congenital or acquired fibrinogen deficiency or Factor XIII deficiency. Cryoprecipitate is not indicated in hemophilia A and von Willebrand disease when virus-inactivated concentrates are available. Because it does not contain clinically significant amounts of other coagulation factors, Cryoprecipitated AHF is not indicated as the sole treatment for DIC, but is an important component in the treatment of disorders with low fibrinogen. Cryoprecipitated AHF has also been reported to be beneficial in treating the bleeding tendency associated with uremia[70]; however, its use should be restricted to those who are unresponsive to nontransfusion therapy (eg, dialysis, desmopressin), because the latter approach is free of the potential infectious complications of Cryoprecipitated AHF.[71] Small amounts of cryoprecipitate (sometimes autologous) are also used as a fibrinogen source and mixed with thrombin to prepare "fibrin sealant" to aid in surgical hemostasis and for other purposes.[72] See Chapter 2: Plasma Derivatives.

Contraindications and Precautions

Cryoprecipitated AHF should not be used to treat patients with deficiencies of factors other than fibrinogen or Factor XIII. ABO-compatible cryoprecipitate is not required due to the small amount of plasma, although this volume of plasma may be clinically significant in infants. In rare instances, infusion of large amounts of ABO-incompatible units of Cryoprecipitated AHF can cause hemolysis; a positive DAT can be seen with infusion of smaller doses. The risk of infectious disease transmission, for each unit of Cryoprecipitated AHF given, is the same as that for FFP.

Dose and Administration

Before infusion, the cryoprecipitate is thawed at 30 to 37 C. Each unit will increase fibrinogen by 5 to 10 mg/dL in an average-size adult. The hemostatic level is ≥ 100 mg/dL fibrinogen. Concentrates are administered through a blood administration set with a 180- to 250-micron filter; no compatibility test is required. If a single unit of Cryoprecipitated AHF Thawed is not used immediately, it may be stored no more than 6 hours at room temperature or no more than 4 hours after pooling.

Oxygen Therapeutics

The availability of oxygen therapeutics (red cell substitutes) remains limited. Modified hemoglobin compounds, perflurocarbon solutions, and lipid encapsulated hemoglobins are the three types of products in development; however, as this book goes to press, none are available outside of clinical trials.[73] Challenges remain in the search for a product that will carry oxygen and deliver it effectively to hypoxic tissues without unacceptable side effects. In the case of cell free hemoglobin preparations, the demonstrated ability of these substances to scavenge nitric oxide may lead to unwanted vasoconstriction. Although perflurocarbons are efficient oxygen carriers, side effects such as thrombocytopenia and flu-like symptoms may limit the infusion volume. Further work is needed to perfect an oxygen delivery system that does not rely on red cells.

Pathogen Reduction

Although the risk of transmission of various pathogens via blood transfusion continues to decrease as a result of improvements in donor screening and laboratory testing, concern remains over the transmission of viruses in the "window period " of infection, as well as the transmission of other pathogenic organsisms, such as bacteria, protozoa, or other viruses for which routine testing is not available. In addition, it is not possible to test for the presence of infection with an agent before it has been identified. The emergence of HIV as a catastrophic entity transmitted by blood transfusion could not have been anticipated, and should serve to remind us of the changing nature of blood safety. Because of these limitations, recent efforts have focused on developing technologies that treat blood components to eliminate contaminating pathogens without the need to specifically test for their presence. Although pathogen inactivation is an attractive prospect, it is essential that the safety and efficacy of the treated product are not compromised. Thus far, the addition of a solvent and detergent to eliminate enveloped viruses has been licensed by FDA for use in plasma and some plasma derivatives.[74] Other technologies include the use of photoactivated psoralens,[75] which has been investigated for use in platelet and plasma components. S303,™ Inactine,™ and riboflavin are novel compounds for pathogen reduction of red cell components. These compounds all interfere with DNA and RNA replication.[76]

References

1. Gorlin JB, ed. Standards for blood banks and transfusion services, 21st ed. Bethesda, MD: American Association of Blood Banks, 2002.
2. Moore GL, Ledford ME, Peck CC. The in vitro evaluation of modifications in CPD-adenine anticoagulated-preserved blood at various hematocrits. Transfusion 1980;20: 419-26.
3. Heaton A, Miripol J, Aster R, et al. Use of Adsol preservation solution for prolonged storage of low viscosity AS-1 red blood cells. Br J Haematol 1984;57:467-78.
4. Simon TL, Marcus CS, Myhre BA, Nelson EJ. Effects of AS-3 nutrient-additive solution on 42 and 49 days of storage of red cells. Transfusion 1987;27:178-82.
5. Welch HG, Meehan KR, Goodnough LT. Prudent strategies for elective red blood cell transfusion. Ann Intern Med 1992;116:393-402.
6. Meryman HT, Hornblower M. The preparation of red cells depleted of leukocytes. Transfusion 1986;26:101-6.
7. Sirchia G, Rebulla P, Parravicini A, et al. Leukocyte depletion of red cell units at the bedside by transfusion through a new filter. Transfusion 1987;27:402-5.
8. Rebulla P, Porretti L, Bertolini F, et al. White cell-reduced red cells prepared by filtration: A critical evaluation of current filters and methods for counting residual white cells. Transfusion 1993;33:128-33.
9. Pietersz RN, Steneker I, Reesink HW. Prestorage leukocyte depletion of blood products in a closed system. Transfus Med Rev 1993;7:17-24.

10. Lane TA, Anderson KC, Goodnough LT, et al. Leukocyte reduction in blood component therapy. Ann Intern Med 1992;117:151-62.

11. Stack G, Snyder EL. Cytokine generation in stored platelet concentrates. Transfusion 1994;34:20-5.

12. Stack G, Baril L, Napychank P, Snyder EL. Cytokine generation in stored, white-cell-reduced, and bacterially contaminated units of red cells. Transfusion 1995;35:199-203.

13. Pomper GJ, Chai L, Champion MH, et al. Incidence of febrile and allergic reactions following introduction of pre-storage universal leukoreduction of random donor platelets and red cells. Tranfsusion 2001;41(suppl):111S.

14. Claas FHJ, Smeenk RJT, Schmidt R, et al. Allo-immunization against the MHC antigens after platelet transfusions is due to contaminating leukocytes in the platelet suspension. Exp Hematol 1981;9:84-9.

15. Perkins HA, Payne R, Ferguson J, Wood M. Non-hemolytic febrile transfusion reactions. Quantitative effects of blood components with emphasis on isoantigenic incompatibility of leukocytes. Vox Sang 1966;11:578-99.

16. TRAP Study Group. Leukocyte reduction and ultraviolet B irradiation of platelets to prevent alloimmunization and refractoriness to platelet transfusions. N Engl J Med 1997; 337:1861-9.

17. Sayers MH, Anderson KC, Goodnough LT, et al. Reducing the risk for transfusion-transmitted cytomegalovirus infection. Ann Intern Med 1992;116:55-62.

18. Bowden RA, Cays MJ, Schoch G, et al. Comparison of filtered blood (FB) to seronegative blood products (SB) for prevention of cytomegalovirus (CMV) infection after marrow transplant. Blood 1995;86:3598-603.

19. Narvios AB, Przepiorka D, Tarrand J, et al. Transfusion support using filtered unscreened blood products for cytomegalovirus-negative allogeneic marrow transplant recipients. Bone Marrow Transplant 1998;22:575-7.

20. Laupacis A, Brown J, Costello B, et al. Prevention of posttransfusion CMV in the era of universal WBC reduction: A concensus statement. Transfusion 2001;41:560-9.

21. Blajchman MA. Allogeneic blood transfusions, immuno-modulation, and postoperative bacterial infection: Do we have the answers yet? (editorial) Transfusion 1997;37: 121-5.

22. Blajchman MA, Dzik WH, Vamvakas EC, et al. Clinical and molecular basis of transfusion-induced immunomo-dulation:summary of the proceedings of a state-of-the-art conference. Transfus Med Rev 2001;15(2):108-35.

23. Haugen RK. Hepatitis after the transfusion of frozen red cells and washed red cells. N Engl J Med 1979;301:393-5.

24. Chaplin H. Frozen red cells revisited. N Engl J Med 1984; 311:1696-8.

25. Schiffer CA, Lee EJ, Ness PM, Reilly J. Clinical evalua-tion of platelets stored for one to five days. Blood 1986; 67:1591-4.

26. NIH consensus development conference. Platelet transfu-sion therapy. JAMA 1987;257:1777-80.

27. College of American Pathologists. Practice parameter for the use of fresh-frozen plasma, cryoprecipitate, and plate-lets. JAMA 1994;271:777-81.

28. Gmur J, Burger J, Schanz U, et al. Safety of stringent pro-phylactic platelet transfusion policy for patients with acute leukaemia. Lancet 1991;338:1223-6.

29. Rebulla P, Finazzi G, Marangoni F, et al. The threshold for prophylactic platelet transfusions in adults with acute myeloid leukemia. N Engl J Med 1997;337:1870-5.

30. Heckman KD, Weiner GJ, Davis CS, et al. Randomized study of prophylactic platelet transfusion threshold during induction therapy for adult acute leukemia: 10,000/µL ver-sus 20,000/µL. J Clin Oncol 1997;15:1143-9.

31. Reed RL, Ciavarella D, Heimbach DM, et al. Prophylactic platelet administration during massive transfusion. Ann Surg 1986;203:40-8.

32. Mannucci PM, Federici AB, Sirchia G. Hemostasis testing during massive blood replacement: A study of 172 cases. Vox Sang 1982;42:113-23.

33. Muylle L, Joos M, Wouters E, et al. Increased tumor ne-crosis factor alpha (TNF α), interleukin 1 (IL-1), and

interleukin 6 (IL-6) levels in the plasma of stored platelet concentrates: Relationship between TNF α and IL-6 levels and febrile transfusion reactions. Transfusion 1993;33: 195-9.

34. Heddle NM, Blajchman MA. The leukodepletion of cellular blood products in the prevention of HLA-alloimmunization and refractoriness to allogeneic platelet transfusions. Blood 1995;85:603-6.

35. Pierce RN, Reich LM, Mayer K. Hemolysis following platelet transfusions from ABO-incompatible donors. Transfusion 1985;25:60-2.

36. Blajchman MA, Goldman M. Bacterial contamination of platelet concentrates: Incidence, significance and prevention. Semin Hematol 2001;38(suppl 11):20-6.

37. Yankee RA, Grumet FC, Rogentine GN. Platelet transfusion therapy: The selection of compatible platelet donors for refractory patients by lymphocyte HLA typing. N Engl J Med 1969;281:1208-12.

38. Bishop JF, McGrath K, Wolf MM, et al. Clinical factors influencing the efficacy of pooled platelet transfusions. Blood 1988;71:383-7.

39. Kickler TS, Braine HG, Ness PM, et al. A radiolabeled antiglobulin test for crossmatching platelet transfusions. Blood 1983;61:238-42.

40. Daly PA, Schiffer CA, Aisner J, Wiernik PH. Platelet transfusion therapy: One-hour posttransfusion increments are valuable in predicting the need for HLA-matched preparations. JAMA 1980;243:435-8.

41. Ness P, Braine H, King K, et al. Single-donor platelets reduce the risk of septic platelet transfusion reactions. Transfusion 2001;41:857-61.

42. Larsson LG, Welsh VJ, Ladd DJ. Acute intravascular hemolysis secondary to out-of-group platelet transfusion. Transfusion 2000;40:902-6.

43. Menitove JE, McElligott MC, Aster RH. Febrile transfusion reaction: What blood component should be given next? Vox Sang 1982;42:318-21.

44. Sniecinski MR, ODonnell B, Norwicki B, Hill LR. Prevention of refractoriness and HLA-alloimmunization using filtered blood products. Blood 1988;71:1402-7.

45. Andreu J, Dewailly C, Leberre MC, et al. Prevention of HLA immunization with leukocyte-poor packed red cells and platelet concentrates obtained by filtration. Blood 1988;72:964-9.

46. Bertholf MF, Mintz PD. Comparison of plateletpheresis using two cell separators and identical donors. Transfusion 1989;29:521-3.

47. Anderson KC, Gorgone BC, Wahlers E, et al. Preparation and utilization of leukocyte poor apheresis platelets. Transfus Sci 1991;12:163-70.

48. Slichter SJ. Platelet transfusion therapy. Hematol Oncol Clin North Am 1990;4:291-311.

49. Heddle NM, Klama L, Singer J, et al. The role of plasma in platelet concentrates in transfusion reactions. N Engl J Med 1994;331:625-8.

50. Aye MT, Palmer DS, Giulivi A, Hashemi S. Effect of filtration of platelet concentrates on the accumulation of cytokines and platelet release factors during storage. Transfusion 1995;35:117-24.

51. Ferrara JL. The febrile platelet transfusion reaction: A cytokine shower. Transfusion 1995;35:89-90.

52. Strauss RG, Rohret PA, Randels MJ, Winegarden DC. Granulocyte collection. J Clin Apheresis 1991;6:241-3.

53. Dale DC, Liles WC, Llewellyn C, et al. Neutrophil transfusions: Kinetics and functions of neutrophils mobilized with granulocyte colony-stimulating factor and dexamethasone. Transfusion 1998;38:713-21.

54. Jendiroba DB, Lichtiger B, Anaissie E, et al. Evaluation and comparison of three mobilization methods for the collection of granulocytes. Transfusion 1998;38:722-8.

55. Stroncek DF, Clay ME, Petzoldt ML, et al. Treatment of normal individuals with granulocyte colony-stimulating factor: Donor experiences and the effects on peripheral blood CD34+ cell counts and on the collection of peripheral blood stem cells. Transfusion 1996;36:601-10.

56. Adkins D, Spitzer G, Johnston M, et al. Transfusions of granulocyte colony-stimulating factor-mobilized granulocyte components to allogeneic transplant recipients: Analysis of kinetics and factors determining posttransfusion neutrophil and platelet counts. Transfusion 1997;37: 737-48.

57. Lane TA. Granulocyte storage. Transfus Med Rev 1990; 4:23-34.

58. Cairo MS. The use of granulocyte transfusion in neonatal sepsis. Transfus Med Rev 1990;4:14-22.

59. Strauss RG, Connett JE, Gale RP, et al. A controlled trial of prophylactic granulocyte transfusions during initial induction chemotherapy for acute myelogenous leukemia. N Engl J Med 1981;305:597-603.

60. Strauss R. Neutrophil (granulocyte) transfusions in the new millennium (editorial). Transfusion 1998;38:710-2.

61. Vamvakas EC, Pineda AA. Meta-analysis of clinical studies of the efficacy of granulocytes transfusions in the treatment of bacterial sepsis. J Clin Apheresis 1996;11:1-9.

62. Dutcher JP, Kendall J, Norris D, et al. Granulocyte transfusion therapy and amphotericin B: Adverse reactions? Am J Hematol 1989;31:102-8.

63. Dutcher JP. Granulocyte transfusion therapy. Am J Med Sci 1984;287:11-7.

64. Nilsson L, Hedner U, Nilsson M, et al. Shelf-life of bank blood and stored plasma with special reference to coagulation factors. Transfusion 1983;23:377-81.

65. Horowitz B, Bonomo R, Prince AM, et al. Solvent/detergent-treated plasma: A virus-inactivated substitute for fresh frozen plasma. Blood 1992;79:826-31.

66. NIH consensus development conference. Fresh frozen plasma: Indications and risks. JAMA 1985;253:551-3.

67. Rock G, Shuman KH, Sutton DM, et al. Cryosupernatant as replacement fluid for plasma exchange in thrombotic thrombocytopenic purpura. Members of the Canadian Apheresis Group. Br J Haematol 1996;94:383-6.

68. Bowden R, Sayers M. The risk of transmitting cytomegalovirus infection by fresh frozen plasma. Transfusion 1990;30:762-3.

69. Braunstein AH, Oberman HA. Transfusion of plasma components. Transfusion 1984;24:281-6.
70. Janson PA, Jubelirer SJ, Weinstein MJ, Deykin D. Treatment of the bleeding tendency in uremia with cryoprecipitate. N Engl J Med 1980;303:1318-22.
71. Remuzzi G. Bleeding in renal failure. Lancet 1988;1: 1205-8.
72. Gibble JW, Ness PM. Fibrin glue: The perfect operative sealant? Transfusion 1990;30:741-7.
73. Winslow R. New transfusion strategies: Red cell substitutes. Annu Rev Med 1999;50:337-53.
74. Klein HG, Dodd RY, Dzik WH, et al. Current status of solvent-detergent treated frozen plasma. Transfusion 1998; 38:102-7.
75. Lin L, Cook DN, Wiesehahn GP, et al. Photochemical inactivation of viruses and bacteria in platelet concentrates by use of a novel psoralen and long-wavelength ultraviolet light. Transfusion 1997;37:423-35.
76. AuBuchon JP, Pickard CA, Herschel LH, et al. Production of pathogen-inactivated RBC concentrates using PEN110 chemistry: A Phase I clinical study. Transfusion 2002; 42:146-52.

Factor VIII Concentrate

Description of Products

Factor VIII preparations can be derived from human plasma or produced by recombinant technology. Recombinant Factor VIII is produced in established hamster cell lines, and is stabilized with the addition of human albumin. Because it is thought to be extraordinarily safe in regard to transmitting human infectious organisms, it has become the product of choice for treating patients with hemophilia A, particularly young and newly diagnosed patients who have never been exposed to human-derived Factor VIII concentrates. Recently, recombinant Factor VIII products without the addition of albumin as a stabilizer have come onto the market.[1,2] This includes a recombinant Factor VIII product that lacks the B domain and was recently licensed in the United States. Human plasma-derived Factor VIII concentrate [also referred to as antihemophilic factor (AHF)] is prepared by fractionation of pooled human plasma that is frozen soon after phlebotomy. Several types of human plasma-derived Factor VIII concentrate are available. All products take the form of a sterile, stable, lyophilized concentrate. They differ in terms of protein purity and the method used to inactivate viruses. The purity is usually expressed by the specific activity, which refers to units of clotting factor per milligram of protein. Factor VIII concentrate has the advantage of providing a product with known dosage and small volume.

The purest products are produced through immunoaffinity chromatography using murine monoclonal antibodies to a portion of the Factor VIII complex.[3,4] The purity of these products is greater than 90% before the addition of albumin, which is used as a stabilizer.

Various procedures are used to inactivate viruses in Factor VIII products and reduce the risk of infectious disease transmission.[5,6] These methods include a combination of pasteurization and solvent/detergent treatment, and affinity chromatography preparation. None of the currently available Factor VIII concentrates have been associated with transmission of human immunodeficiency virus (HIV). However, it should be noted that no treatment procedure or combination of procedures completely eliminates the risk of virus transmission. This may be particularly relevant with respect to certain non-lipid-enveloped viruses such as hepatitis A and parvovirus B19.[7,8] A half-life range of 12 to 18 hours has been reported for all Factor VIII products. However, active bleeding or inhibitor development (antibodies directed against the coagulation factor) may reduce the half-life.

Indications

Factor VIII concentrate is indicated for the treatment or prevention of bleeding episodes in hemophilia A patients with moderate-to-severe congenital Factor VIII deficiency and for patients with low-titer Factor VIII inhibitors when levels do not exceed 5 to 10 Bethesda units/mL. When Factor VIII concentrate is used for patients with inhibitors, frequent laboratory assays of Factor VIII levels should be performed. Certain Factor VIII concentrates (eg, Humate-P, Alphanate, Koate DVI) have been successfully used to treat von Willebrand disease because they contain the von Willebrand factor (vWF) needed for normal platelet function.[1,9] These products are virus-inactivated and have become the product of choice to treat von Willebrand disease when clinically appropriate. Cryoprecipitate should not be used to treat von Willebrand disease except in emergency situations when these concentrates are not available.

Contraindications and Precautions

Approximately 10% to 15% of individuals with severe hemophilia receiving plasma-derived Factor VIII develop Factor VIII inhibitors. Hemophiliacs previously treated with plasma-derived Factor VIII concentrates do not seem to develop inhibitors any more frequently than those treated with recombinant Factor VIII.[10]

Dose and Administration

The quantity of Factor VIII coagulant activity is stated on the bottle in terms of international units (IU). One IU is the amount of Factor VIII coagulant activity present in 1 mL of normal plasma. Initial doses to achieve levels of 30% to 100% (depending on the clinical circumstance) are calculated using the following formula:

$$\text{Plasma volume (PV, mL)} = 40 \text{ mL/kg} \times \text{body weight (kg)}$$

$$\text{Desired units of Factor VIII} = \frac{\text{PV} \times [\text{desired level (\%)} - \text{initial level (\%)}]}{100}$$

An alternative method of calculation is that each unit of Factor VIII infused per kilogram of body weight yields a 2% rise in the plasma Factor VIII level (ie, 0.02 IU/mL).

Factor VIII concentrates are prepared in lyophilized form and are reconstituted aseptically with a sterile diluent provided by the manufacturer. They must be filtered before administration either by using an infusion set with a standard blood filter or by reconstituting the concentrate using a filter needle provided with the product. Cryoprecipitate should not be used as an alternative to recombinant or human-derived Factor VIII concentrates as it has a higher risk of transmitting infectious agents.[1] Once a loading dose of a Factor VIII preparation is given, subsequent dosing at 50% of the loading dose is usually given by intravenous bolus infusion every 8 to 12 hours. An alternate method of administration is continuous infusion.[11] The duration of treatment depends on the patients response and the severity of bleeding. Hospitalized patients who require repeated doses or infusions should be monitored with Factor VIII levels to ensure adequate replacement. When Factor VIII is used for treatment of patients with low level Factor VIII inhibitors, effectiveness of therapy should be assessed both by monitoring Factor VIII levels and inhibitor titers. Reconstituted Factor VIII should be used as quickly as possible, although the shelf life after reconstitution will depend on the type of Factor VIII concentrate used.

Factor IX Concentrates

Description of Products

Recombinant and plasma-derived Factor IX concentrates are available.[12] Recombinant Factor IX concentrate is produced in a Chinese hamster ovary cell line. Because no human products are used, it is not thought to transmit human infectious diseases. For this reason, recombinant Factor IX is the treatment of choice for new patients with hemophilia B and for those with limited exposure to human-derived Factor IX products.[1] Coagulation Factor IX is a highly purified preparation containing trace amounts (nontherapeutic) of Factors II, VII, and X. These concentrates were developed by advanced chromatographic methods or monoclonal antibody purification in order to provide a less thrombogenic material. Factor IX Complex (prothrombin complex) is a crude preparation that contains in addition to Factor IX, some quantities of Factors II, VII, and X, some of which may be activated. Human-derived Factor IX concentrates are now heat-treated, solvent/detergent-treated, or produced using recombinant technology to decrease the risk of hepatitis, HIV, and other viral diseases.[5] However, no procedure completely eliminates the risk of transmission of viral diseases. The half-life of Factor IX products in Factor-IX-deficient patients has been reported to range from 18 to 32 hours.[13]

Indications

Factor IX Deficiency

Factor IX concentrates are used for the treatment of patients with Factor IX deficiency, commonly known as hemophilia B.

Treatment of Factor Inhibitors

Patients with inhibitors may be treated with Factor IX Complex concentrates, which contain Factor VIII inhibitor bypass activity. These fractionated, pooled human plasma products also contain activated vitamin-K-dependent factors. They have been used to treat both hemophiliacs and nonhemophiliacs with factor inhibitors.[1] A porcine Factor VIII material for treatment of hemophilia A patients with Factor VIII inhibitors is also available.[14] This concentrate has not undergone any process of virus inactivation, but it has been screened for porcine viruses. It has not been shown to transmit infections to humans. Recombinant Factor VIIa is used to treat patients with hemophilia who have developed inhibitors.[15,16] The appropriate dose of this product is debated, and patients may require frequent doses to control bleeding. Because none of the products are universally effective, consultation with a physician experienced in their use is advised.[17]

Contraindications and Precautions

Factor IX Complex should be used with caution in patients with liver disease. There have been reports of thrombosis and disseminated intravascular coagulation (DIC) associated with the use of these concentrates in patients with presumed deficiencies of antithrombin (particularly patients with liver disease). The etiology of this complication may relate to the presence of activated factors and diminished hepatic clearance, leading to the accumulation of high levels of the factors. Patients with inhibitors to Factor VIII who have been treated with high doses of Factor IX Complex have developed acute myocardial infarction caused by transmural hemorrhage rather than demonstrable thrombosis.[18] Coagulation Factor IX concentrates appear to be substantially less thrombogenic than Factor IX Complex preparations. Side effects associated with rapid infusion of Factor IX Complex include chills, fever, headache, nausea, and flushing. Rapid administration of coagulation Factor IX may also produce vasomotor reactions. Recombinant Factor VIIa appears to have a lower risk of thrombotic complications when compared with the Factor IX Complex concentrates.

Dose and Administration

The quantity of Factor IX is stated on the bottle in terms of activity units. One unit of Factor IX activity is equivalent to that found in 1mL of normal human plasma. The dose required depends on the clinical symptoms and needs of the patient. The amount of Factor IX concentrate to infuse is calculated using the same formula as that used for Factor VIII dosing. However, the in-vivo recovery is only approximately 50% because of extravascular distribution. Thus, each unit of Factor IX infused per kilogram of body weight will yield a 1% rise in the circulating Factor IX level (ie, approximately half that of Factor VIII). Some physicians compensate for the low recovery by doubling the loading dose. Repeat doses of Factor IX should be half of the loading dose administered every 18 to 24 hours. Recent reports suggest that Factor IX, like Factor VIII, can also be administered successfully by continuous infusion.[19,20] Factor IX concentrates should be aseptically reconstituted with the sterile diluent provided by the manufacturer. Reconstituted material must be filtered before use. It should be infused intravenously as soon as possible after reconstitution, within the time limit established for a particular product.

Other Recombinant and Plasma Protein Derivatives

Antithrombin Concentrate

Antithrombin (AT) is an important inhibitor of coagulation. Thrombin and activated Factors IX, X, XI, and XII are inhibited by AT. The rate at which these factors are inhibited is dramatically increased in the presence of heparin. Congenital deficiencies of AT are associated with thrombotic disease.[21] AT concentrates are used to treat patients with hereditary AT deficiency (where plasma levels are approximately 50% of that in normal plasma) who have thrombosis or require prophylaxis when they are scheduled to undergo surgical or obstetric procedures. The efficacy of AT concentrates in acquired AT deficiency (eg, due to heparin resistance or DIC) remains unproven.[22,23] AT concentrates are prepared from pooled human plasma and are heat-treated to reduce the risk of virus transmission.

Recombinant Factor VIIa

Recombinant Factor VIIa is a recently licensed product to treat bleeding in hemophilia patients who have an inhibitor and to treat patients who have developed an acquired inhibitor to Factor VIII. The exact mechanism of action of recombinant Factor VIIa is not fully known but probably works by enhancing thrombin generation through direct activation of Factor X, leading to increased thrombin-activated platelet surfaces. Although not licensed for such, recombinant Factor VIIa has been used to treat bleeding in many other clinical situations including trauma patients, and those with liver disease or Glanzmann's thrombasthenia. The most appropriate dose for treating any indication is still not fully established. Thrombosis is a risk, but it appears to be low.[15,16]

Protein C Concentrate

Protein C is another important inhibitor of coagulation. It is a vitamin-K-dependent factor that is converted to its active form by the thrombin/thrombomodulin complex. Activated protein C, in the presence of protein S, is a potent inhibitor of the activated forms of Factors V and VIII. Heterozygous protein C deficiency is associated with an increased risk of recurrent venous thrombosis. Homozygous deficiency results in a severe thrombotic disorder in the newborn period manifested as purpura fulminans and DIC. Protein C can be found in Factor IX Complex, but this product is contraindicated in protein C deficiency states because of the risk of thrombosis. Investigational protein C concentrates have been used successfully and are undergoing clinical evaluation.[24] A new, recently licensed recombinant human-activated protein C concentrate was shown to have efficacy in treating patients with severe sepsis and a high risk of mortality.[25]

C1-Esterase Inhibitor

C1-esterase inhibitor (C1-INH) is an important regulator of the complement cascade. A deficiency of this protein is associated with hereditary angioedema, an autosomal-dominant disease characterized by episodic swelling of respiratory and gastrointestinal mucosa and submucosa.[26] Acute upper-airway obstruction secondary to soft tissue edema is a major cause of mortality in these patients. Fresh frozen plasma has been used as replacement therapy for acute episodes or surgical prophylaxis, but efficacy is limited by the volumes needed and the delay caused by thawing. Virus-inactivated C1-INH concentrates have been used in Europe for several years, but no preparations are approved for use in the United States.[27]

Alpha₁-Proteinase Inhibitor

Alpha$_1$-proteinase inhibitor (API, also known as alpha$_1$-antitrypsin) is a serine proteinase inhibitor of neutrophil elastase. API deficiency is associated with pulmonary emphysema and liver disease.[28] API concentrate is licensed by the Food and Drug Administration (FDA) as a product prepared from pooled human plasma and is virus-inactivated using heat treatment. API concentrate is used intravenously for long-term therapy in patients with severe API deficiency and clinically demonstrable panacinar emphysema.[29] An aerosol form of API is currently under clinical evaluation.

Fibrin Sealant

Cryoprecipitated AHF has been used as a source of fibrinogen for the preparation of a surgical tissue sealant or biological glue. One or two units of autologous or allogeneic Cryoprecipitated AHF are mixed with a source of thrombin and calcium chloride and applied to a surgical site to generate a crosslinked fibrin clot to stem bleeding.[30] Although there have been no reported cases of viral disease transmission with the use of these preparations, the FDA has licensed a fibrin sealant kit that uses lyophilized, virus-inactivated, pooled human fibrinogen and thrombin with a bovine albumin stabilizer. The kit has the benefit of standardization of preparation and ease of administration.[31] Of note, homemade fibrin sealants have used bovine thrombin preparations that contain bovine Factor V. A number of patients have made antibodies to the bovine Factor V, resulting in serious clinical sequelae.[32]

Factor XIII Concentrate

Fibrogammin P is a plasma-derived Factor XIII concentrate used to treat patients with Factor XIII deficiency. It is not yet licensed in the United States and is only available on a research basis.[1]

Albumin and Plasma Protein Fraction

Description of Product

Albumin is derived from donor plasma obtained from whole blood or through plasmapheresis. It is composed of 96% albumin and 4% globulin and other proteins and is prepared by the cold alcohol fractionation process. These derivatives are subsequently heated to 60 C for 10 hours. Because of this treatment, these products do not transmit viral diseases. Plasma protein fraction (PPF) is a similar product, except that it is subjected to fewer purification steps in the fractionation process. PPF contains about 83% albumin and 17% globulin. Normal serum albumin is available as a 25% or a 5% solution, while PPF is available as a 5% solution. Each has a sodium content of about 145 mmol/L (145 mEq/L). The 5% albumin solution is osmotically and oncotically equivalent to plasma, while the 25% solution is osmotically and oncotically five times greater than that of plasma. Albumin has a plasma half-life of 16 hours. These products can be stored up to 5 years at 2 to 10 C.

Indications

Albumin is used for its oncotic activity in patients who are both hypovolemic and hypoproteinemic (eg, clinical settings of shock, thermal injury, and the nephrotic syndrome).[33,34] However, the specific clinical situations for which albumin therapy is recommended and has proved to be beneficial remain controversial. A recent meta-analysis of the available medical literature suggests that albumin may be harmful to critically ill patients in comparison with the use of crystalloids or no albumin.[35] This finding was recently challenged in a newly published review that supported the safety of albumin.[36] Additional controlled trials on the use of albumin are warranted. Indications for the use of PPF parallel those given for 5% albumin.

Contraindications and Precautions

Use of the 25% albumin solution is contraindicated in dehydrated patients unless it is supplemented by the infusion of crystalloid solutions to provide volume expansion. The 25% albumin solution can be diluted only with normal saline or D5W. Sterile water should not be used.[37,38] Both albumin and PPF should be used with caution in patients who are susceptible to fluid overload. Reported side effects include flushing, urticaria, chills, fever, and headache. Rapid infusion of PPF at rates higher than 10 mL/minute has produced hypotension attributed to the presence of both sodium acetate and Hageman factor fragments.[39] PPF, but not albumin, is contraindicated for intra-arterial administration or infusion during cardiopulmonary bypass. Albumin and PPF have not been reported to transmit viruses, although investigations regarding prior transmission are ongoing.

Dose and Administration

Albumin and PPF need not be given through a filter. Treatment of hypotension with albumin and PPF should be guided by the patients hemodynamic response. A 500-mL dose (10-20 mL/kg in children) is given rapidly for shock. In the absence of symptomatic hypovolemia, an infusion rate of 1 to 2 mL/minute is suitable. Rate restrictions do apply to the infusion of PPF (see above). In burn patients, the dose of albumin or PPF is the amount necessary to maintain the circulating plasma protein level at 5.2 g/dL or higher.

Albumin will not correct chronic hypoalbuminemia and should not be used for long-term therapy.[34]

Synthetic Volume Expanders

Description of Products

Crystalloid solutions such as normal saline and Ringer's lactate are isotonic and isosmotic with plasma. Normal saline contains only sodium and chloride ions, while Ringer's lactate also contains potassium, calcium, and lactate. Hypotonic solutions of sodium chloride are also available.

Colloids used for volume expansion include Dextran and hydroxyethyl starch (HES). Dextrans are branched-chain polysaccharides composed of glucose units. They are available in a low-molecular-weight (Dextran 40) and a high-molecular-weight (Dextran 70) form and are prepared as a 6% or 10% solution in dextrose or saline, respectively. The half-life of Dextran is approximately 6 hours. HES is available as a 6% solution in normal saline. The intravascular half-life of HES is greater than 24 hours.

Indications

By virtue of their oncotic properties, both Dextran and HES are useful as volume expanders in hemorrhagic shock and the treatment of burns. Crystalloid solutions alone expand the plasma volume temporarily as they rapidly cross capillary membranes with only one-third of the salt solution remaining in the intravascular space.[40] Accordingly, two to three volumes of crystalloid are required to replace one volume of lost plasma. However, crystalloid solutions are useful in patients who are in shock resulting from hemorrhage or burns in whom it is necessary to rapidly expand the plasma volume.[34] For burn patients, crystalloid is the treatment of choice for volume expansion in the first 24 hours, because the capillary leak in the burned areas renders albumin ineffective as an oncotic agent. Crystalloid solutions, Dextran, and HES are relatively nontoxic and inexpensive, are readily available, can be stored at room temperature, require no compatibility testing, and are free of the risk of transfusion-transmitted disease. The relative merits of crystalloid vs colloid solutions for acute hypovolemia remain controversial.[34,41]

Contraindications and Precautions

Dextran can produce anaphylactic reactions, fever, rash, tachycardia, and hypotension. Because of Dextran's interference with platelet function and its stimulation of fibrinolysis, its use is associated with increased bleeding tendencies. Renal failure has also been reported with infusion of the low-molecular-weight products. Dextran may also interfere with blood typing and crossmatching. The side effects associated with HES occur less frequently than those reported for Dextran, but do include prolongation of prothrombin time and partial thromboplastin time as well as pruritus. All volume expanders require consideration of the possibility of fluid overload.

Administration

Crystalloid solutions, Dextran, and HES do not have to be administered through a blood filter.

Immune Globulin

Description of Products

Immune Globulins are prepared by cold ethanol fractionation from pools of human plasma. Gammaglobulin preparations and specific hyperimmune globulin preparations with high titers against specific infectious agents or toxins are available for intramuscular use (IMIG). These products have a number of disadvantages: IM administration requires 4-7 days to achieve effective plasma levels; the maximum dose that can be given is limited by muscle mass; administration may be painful; and IMIG can undergo proteolytic breakdown at the IM site.[42] Intramuscular products are now given primarily for disease prophylaxis. These preparations are sterile solutions with protein concentrations of approximately 16.5 g/dL. The predominant immunoglobulin is IgG, but IgA and IgM may also be present.

Intravenous gammaglobulin (IVIG) preparations minimize some of the disadvantages of IMIG. Sterile, lyophilized IVIG preparations differ in mode of preparation, use of additives, pH, and their protein content (stated on the vial).[42,43] More than 90% of the protein is IgG; there are only trace quantities of IgA and IgM. IVIG products provide a way of achieving peak levels of IgG immediately after infusion. The gammaglobulin molecules of IVIG preparations are intact. The half-lives of IVIG and IMIG preparations vary from 18 to 32 days, the same as that of native IgG.[42]

Indications

Immune Globulin preparations can be used to provide passive antibody prophylaxis for susceptible individuals exposed to certain diseases and as replacement therapy in primary immunodeficiency states (eg, common variable immunodeficiency, Wiskott-Aldrich syndrome, severe combined immunodeficiency).[42,44,45] IVIG can be used as an immunomodulating agent to treat selected patients with autoimmune disorders such as acute and chronic idiopathic thrombocytopenic purpura (ITP) in children and adults.[46,47] These preparations are also used to treat HIV-related thrombocytopenia, posttransfusion purpura, neonatal alloimmune thrombocytopenia and Guillain-Barré syndrome. They may have utility in treating infection and providing graft-vs-host disease prophylaxis in marrow recipients.[46] The efficacy of IVIG in various clinical settings was assessed in 1990 at a National Institutes of Health Consensus Conference, and further reviews of off-label use and use in autoimmune and inflammatory diseases have been published.[45,48,49]

Contraindications and Precautions

Adverse reactions to Immune Globulin preparations include headache, fatigue, chills, backache, lightheadedness, fever, flushing, and nausea.[50] Individuals with a history of IgA deficiency (with anti-IgA) or severe anaphylactic reactions to plasma products should not, in general, receive Immune Globulin. IM preparations must not be given intravenously because they contain immunoglobulin aggregates that may activate the complement and kinin systems. Immediate hypersensitivity and anaphylactic reactions may then occur. Certain preparations contain very small quantities of IgA. While currently available gammaglobulin products appear to be safe with respect to HIV and hepatitis B transmission, hepatitis C transmission has been observed following the use of some preparations of IVIG.[47,51,52] As a result, solvent/detergent-treated IVIG preparations, free of hepatitis C transmission, have been developed. Passive transfer of ABO and other blood group allo-antibodies may produce a positive direct antiglobulin test result in recipients. Clinically significant hemolysis may occur on rare occasions.[53,54]

Dose and Administration

The dose of Immune Globulin is dependent on the reason for administration, patient characteristics, and the preparation used (IM or IV). Careful attention to the package insert for rate of infusion should be stringently followed, as some data suggest that too rapid an infusion may increase risk of renal abnormality and thrombosis.

Rh Immune Globulin

Description of Product

Rh Immune Globulin (RhIG) is prepared from pooled human plasma. It predominantly contains IgG anti-D. Two dosages are available for either IM or IV administration. A solvent/detergent-treated IV preparation (300-μg and 120-μg doses) is FDA-approved for both suppression of immunization to the D antigen and for treatment of ITP. IM RhIG is available in 300-μg and 50-μg (microdose) forms. A dose of 300 μg of either IM or IV RhIG will protect against the immunizing effect of up to 15 mL of D-positive red cells. These preparations appear to be very safe with respect to infectious disease transmission. There have been no reports of HIV transmission with the use of RhIG.[55,56]

Indications and Dosage

Antepartum

For D-negative females, a 50-μg dose of IM RhIG is protective for abortion, miscarriage, or termination of ectopic pregnancy occurring during the first 12 weeks of gestation (fetal red cell mass at 12 weeks of gestation is estimated to be <2.5 mL). After 12 weeks of gestation, a full dose of IM RhIG should be administered for these indications. A full dose is also recommended for use after amniocentesis.[57-59] Guidelines for IV RhIG use call for a 300-μg dose if amniocentesis or chorionic villus sampling is performed before 34 weeks of gestation. A 120-μg dose of IV RhIG is recommended after termination of pregnancy and following amniocentesis or other obstetric manipulations after 34 weeks of gestation. RhIG should be given (preferably) within 72 hours of performing amniocentesis or any other procedure that may cause fetomaternal hemorrhage (FMH), including termination of pregnancy, unless it has been determined that either the fetus is D negative or that maternal immunization to the D antigen has already occurred. If repeated amnioenteses are performed, additional doses should be considered, particularly if the procedures are performed more than 21 days apart.

Nonimmunized D-negative females should receive antepartum prophylaxis (300 μg) of either IM or IV RhIG at 28 weeks of gestation. This has reduced the number of D-negative females who become immunized during gestation by about 90%.[57]

Postpartum

All D-negative females who deliver D-positive infants should receive a 300-μg dose of IM RhIG or a 120-μg dose of IV RhIG unless previous maternal immunization to the D antigen, not related to antepartum RhIG therapy, has been demonstrated. If the result of the infants typing is questionable, RhIG should be given to the mother. A postpartum maternal blood sample must be drawn, preferably within 1 hour of delivery, and evaluated for the extent of FMH. If the screening test for FMH is positive, hemorrhage must be quantified to assess the need for additional doses of RhIG. This is usually done by performing a Kleihauer-Betke test or a flow cytometric assay. A full dose (300 μg) of IM RhIG protects against alloimmunization to the D antigen after exposure of up to 15 mL of D-positive red cells. In about 1 in 300 deliveries, the FMH exceeds 15 mL of red cells and one or more additional doses of IM RhIG are required. In this setting, IV RhIG may prove to be a convenient alternative compared to multiple IM injections. Additional dosing is required slightly more often when the 120-μg dose of IV RhIG is used because it protects against the immunizing effect of approximately 6 mL of D-positive red cells. There seems to be no risk associated with the administration of excessive amounts of RhIG to D-negative individuals. RhIG should be administered to the mother within 72 hours of delivery. However, if more than 72 hours elapse, the dose should still be given as it may protect against maternal alloimmunization. In addition, RhIG should be administered to a D-negative female when her serum contains blood group antibodies other than anti-D. If antepartum RhIG has been administered, additional postpartum maternal dosing is required if the infant is D-positive. Antepartum administration may cause a positive antibody screen in the mother, but that screen must not be interpreted as active immunization. Antepartum RhIG has been associated with weakly reactive direct antiglobulin test results in the newborn, but this is not associated with clinical evidence of hemolysis.[60] Obtaining a good patient history is essential in determining the likely cause of an anti-D in the pregnant or postpartum female.

Special Considerations

The package insert should be carefully followed for determination of dose for any indication. RhIG may also be used when D-positive blood components are given to D-negative females of childbearing potential and children. A 300-µg IM dose (120-µg IV) is sufficient to protect against the immunizing effect of the D-positive red cells contained in more than 10 units of whole-blood-derived Platelets. Administration of multiple vials of RhIG following the infusion of D-positive red cells to a D-negative recipient has been reported, but this is generally impractical when more than one unit of blood has been transfused. IV RhIG may be more suitable than IM RhIG for this purpose, but the use of either must be weighed against the risk of inducing clinically significant hemolysis in the recipient. In this situation, 20 µg of RhIG should be given within 72 hours for each milliliter of red cells transfused. IV RhIG may also be an important alternative to IM therapy in patients with coagulopathy and significant thrombocytopenia. IV RhIG is approved by the FDA for use in D-positive, non-splenectomized patients with immune thrombocytopenia.[55] The initial dose is 50 µg/kg unless the hemoglobin is less than 10 g/dL, in which case 25 to 40 µg/kg is recommended. Additional doses may be required, depending on the initial response. The primary advantages of IV RhIG over IVIG in the treatment of ITP are its lower cost and lower volume.

References

1. Lusher JM, et al. Medical and Scientific Advisory Council recommendations concerning the treatment of hemophilia and related bleeding disorders. National Hemophilia Foundation, 1999.
2. Schwartz RS, Abildgaard CF, Aledort LM, et al. Human recombinant DNA-derived antihemophilic factor (factor VIII) in the treatment of hemophilia A. Recombinant Factor VIII Study Group. N Engl J Med 1990;323:1800-5.

3. Human factor VIII:C purified using monoclonal antibody to von Willebrand factor. Proceedings from a satellite symposium. Semin Hematol 1988;25(suppl1):1-45.

4. Brettler DB, Forsberg AD, Levine PH, et al. Factor VIII:C concentrate purified from plasma using monoclonal antibodies: Human studies. Blood 1989;73:1859-63.

5. Kasper CK, Lusher JM, and the Transfusion Practices Committee. Recent evolution of clotting factor concentrates for hemophilia A and B. Transfusion 1993;33: 422-34.

6. International Forum. Ways to reduce the risk of transmission of viral infections by plasma and plasma products: A comparison of methods, their advantages and disadvantages. Vox Sang 1988;54:228-45.

7. Soucie JM, Robertson BH, Bell BP, et al. Hepatitis A virus infections associated with clotting factor concentrate in the Unites States. Transfusion 1998;38:573-9.

8. Prowse C, Ludlam CA, Yap PL. Human parvovirus B19 and blood products. Vox Sang 1997;72:1-10.

9. Berntorp E, Nilsson IM. Use of high-purity factor VIII concentrate (Humate-P) in von Willebrand disease. Vox Sang 1989;56:212-7.

10. Bray GL, Gomperts GO, Courter S, et al. A multicenter study of recombinant factor VIII (Recombinate): Safety, efficacy and inhibitor risk in previously untreated patients with hemophilia A. Blood 1994;83:2428-35.

11. Bona RD, Weinstein RA, Weisman SJ, et al. The use of continuous infusion of factor concentrates in the treatment of hemophilia. Am J Hematol 1989;32:8-13.

12. White G, Shapiro A, Ragni M, et al. Clinical evaluation of recombinant factor IX. Semin Hematol 1998;35:33-8.

13. Zauber NP, Levin J. Factor IX levels in patients with hemophilia B (Christmas disease) following transfusion with concentrates of factor IX or fresh frozen plasma (FFP). Medicine 1977;56:213-24.

14. Rubinger M, Houston DS, Schwetz N, et al. Continuous infusion of porcine factor VIII in the management of patients with Factor VIII inhibitors. Am J Hematol 1997;56: 112-8.

15. Hedner U, Glazer S, Pingel K, et al. Successful use of recombinant factor VIIa in patients with severe hemophilia A during synovectomy. Lancet 1988;2:1193.

16. Hedner U, Erhardtsen E. Potential role for rFVIIa in transfusion medicine. Transfusion 2002;42:114-24.

17. Tarantino M, Aledort L. On the treatment of hemorrhage in patients with hemophilia and associated inhibitors (letter). Transfusion 2001;41:1628.

18. Lusher JM. Prediction and management of adverse events associated with the use of factor IX complex concentrates. Semin Hematol 1993;30:36-40.

19. Martinowitz UP, Schulman S. Continuous infusion of factor concentrates: Review of use in hemophilia A and demonstration of safety and efficacy in hemophilia B. Acta Haematol 1995;94:35-42.

20. Menart C, Petit PY, Attali O, et al. Efficacy and safety of continuous infusion of Mononine during five surgical procedures in three hemophilic patients. Am J Hematol 1998; 58:110-6.

21. Menache D, Grossman BJ, Jackson CM. Antithrombin III: Physiology, deficiency and replacement therapy. Transfusion 1992;32:580-8.

22. Fourrier F. Therapeutic applications of antithrombin concentrates in systemic inflammatory disorders. Blood Coagul Fibrinolysis 1998;9:S39-45.

23. Lechner K, Kyrle PA. Antithrombin III concentrates—are they clinically useful? Thromb Haemost 1995;73:340-8.

24. Dreyfus M, Magny JF, Bridey F, et al. Treatment of homozygous protein C deficiency and neonatal purpura fulminans with a purified protein C concentrate. N Engl J Med 1991;325:1565-8.

25. Bernard GR, Vincent J-L, Laterre P-F, et al. Efficacy and safety of recombinant activated protein C for severe sepsis. N Engl J Med 2001;344:699-709.

26. Donald VH, Evans RR. A biochemical abnormality in hereditary angioneurotic edema: Absence of serum inhibitor of C1-esterase. Am J Med 1963;35:37-44.

27. Waytes AT, Rosen FS, Frank MM. Treatment of hereditary angioedema with a vapor-heated C1 inhibitor concentrate. N Engl J Med 1996;334:1630-4.

28. Garver RI Jr, Mornex J-F, Nukiwa T, et al. Alpha$_1$-antitrypsin deficiency and emphysema caused by homozygous inheritance of non-expressing alpha$_1$-antitrypsin genes. N Engl J Med 1986;314:762-6.

29. Wewers MD, Casolaro MA, Sellers SE, et al. Replacement therapy for alpha$_1$-antitrypsin deficiency associated with emphysema. N Engl J Med 1987;316:1055-62.

30. Gibble JW, Ness PM. Fibrin glue: The perfect operative sealant? Transfusion 1990;30:741-7.

31. Martinowitz U, Saltz R. Fibrin sealant. Curr Opin Hematol 1996;3:395-402.

32. Streiff MB, Ness PM. Acquired FV inhibitors: A needless iatrogenic complication of bovine thrombin exposure. Transfusion 2002;42:18-26.

33. Erstad BL, Gales BJ, Rappaport WD. The use of albumin in clinical practice. Arch Intern Med 1991;151:901-11.

34. Vermeulen LC, Ratko TA, Erstad BL, et al. A paradigm for consensus: The University Hospital Consortium guidelines for the use of albumin, nonprotein colloid, and crystalloid solutions. Arch Intern Med 1995;155:373-9.

35. Cochrane Injuries Group Albumin Reviewers. Human albumin administration in critically ill patients: A systematic review of randomised controlled trials. Br Med J 1998; 317:235-40.

36. Wilkes MM, Navackis RJ. Patient survival after human albumin administration—a meta-analysis of randomized, controlled trials. Ann Intern Med 2001;135:149-64.

37. Centers for Disease Control and Prevention. Hemolysis associated with 25% human albumin diluted with sterile water—United States, 1994-1998. Morb Mortal Wkly Rep MMWR 1999;48:157-9.

38. Pierce LR, Gaines A, Varricchio F, Epstein J. Hemolysis and renal failure associated with use of sterile water for injection to dilute 25% albumin solution (letter). Am J Health Supt Pharm 1998;55:1057, 1062, 1070.

39. Olinger GN, Werner PH, Boncheck LI, et al. Vasodilator effects of the sodium acetate in pooled protein fraction. Ann Surg 1979;190:305-11.

40. Cervera AL, Moss G. Crystalloid distribution following hemorrhage and hemodilution: Mathematical model and prediction of optimum volumes for equilibration at normovolemia. J Trauma 1974;14:506-20.

41. Moss GS, Gould S. Plasma expanders—an update. Surg Pharmacol 1988;155:425-37.

42. Berkman SA, Lee ML, Gale RP. Clinical uses of intravenous immunoglobulins. Semin Hematol 1988;25:140-58.

43. Römer J, Morgenthaler JJ, Scherz R, et al. Characterization of various immunoglobulin preparations for intravenous application 1. Protein composition and antibody content. Vox Sang 1982;42:62-73.

44. Boshkov LK, Kelton JG. Use of intravenous gamma globulin as an immune replacement and an immune suppressant. Transfus Med Rev 1989;3:82-120.

45. NIH consensus development conference. Intravenous immunoglobulin: Prevention and treatment of disease. JAMA 1990;264:3189-93.

46. Nydegger UE. New aspects of immunoglobulin treatment for idiopathic thrombocytopenic purpura. Plasma Ther Transfus Technol 1988;9:83-7.

47. Safety of therapeutic immune globulin preparations with respect to transmission of human T lymphotropic virus type III/LAV infection. Morb Mortal Wkly Rep MMWR 1986;35:231-3.

48. Ratko TA, Burnett DA, Foulke GE, et al. Recommendations for off label use of intravenously administered immunoglobulin preparations. JAMA 1995;273:1865-70.

49. MacKay IR, Rosen FS, Kazatchkine MD, Kaveri SV. Immunomodulation of autoimmune and inflammatory diseases with intravenous immune globulin. N Engl J Med 2001;345:747-55.

50. Misbah SA, Chapel HM. Adverse effects of intravenous immunoglobulin. Drug Saf 1993;9:254-62.

51. Bussel J, Cunningham-Rundles C, Feldman C, Horowitz B. Transmission of viral infection by preparation of intra-

venous immunoglobulin. Plasma Ther Transfus Technol 1988;9:193-205.

52. Centers for Disease Control. Outbreak of hepatitis C associated with Intravenous Immunoglobulin administration United States, October 1993-June 1994. Morb Mortal Wkly Rep MMWR 1994;43:505-9.

53. Kim HC, Park CL, Cowan JH, et al. Massive intravascular hemolysis associated with intravenous immunoglobulin in bone marrow transplant recipients. Am J Pediatr Hematol Oncol 1988;10:69-74.

54. Wilson JR, Bhoopalam H, Fisher M. Hemolytic anemia associated with intravenous immunoglobulin. Muscle Nerve 1997;20:1142-5.

55. Bussel JB, Graziano JN, Kimberly RP, et al. Intravenous anti-D treatment of immune thrombocytopenic purpura: Analysis of efficacy, toxicity, and mechanism of effect. Blood 1991;77:1884-93.

56. Lack of transmission of human immunodeficiency virus through $Rh_o(D)$ immune globulin (human). Morb Mortal Wkly Rep MMWR 1987;36(44):728-9.

57. Bowman JM. Antenatal suppression of Rh alloimmunization. Clin Obstet Gyn 1991;34:296-303.

58. American College of Obstetrics and Gynecology. Prevention of Rho(D) isoimmunization. ACOG Practice Bull 1999;4:1-8.

59. Hartwell EA. Use of Rh immune: ASCP practice parameter. Am J Clin Pathol 1998;110:281-92.

60. Pisciotto P, Gorbants I, Sundra M. Antenatal Rh immunoglobulin—help or hindrance? (letter). Transfusion 1985; 25:88.

TRANSFUSION PRACTICES

Maximum Surgical Blood Order Schedule/Type and Screen

Most healthy adult patients with a normal hemoglobin level who undergo elective surgical procedures do not require blood replacement if there is blood loss of less than 1000 mL, provided that intravascular volume is maintained with crystalloid or colloid solutions. In fact, only a small percentage of all surgical patients actually receive blood transfusions.[1]

The maximum surgical blood order schedule (MSBOS) has been used to reduce pretransfusion testing, to avoid outdating of blood units, and to serve as a guide for autologous blood collection. This schedule can be developed by analyzing blood usage for common elective surgical procedures and comparing the number of red cell units crossmatched to the number of units transfused. Surgical procedures with crossmatch/transfusion (C/T) ratios greater than 2.0 are considered to have an excessive number of units of blood ordered and crossmatched.[2] Because the MSBOS serves as the preoperative blood order for surgical patients, the blood bank can collect and process patient specimens more efficiently. Tracking of the C/T ratio for given procedures may help prevent overordering of blood. The MSBOS varies among institutions and is expected to vary with changes in surgical practice, blood bank techniques, and blood components.

For surgical procedures associated with less than a 10% likelihood of requiring blood transfusions, a type-and-screen procedure instead of a crossmatch is recommended.[1] With a type and screen, the transfusion service determines the patient's ABO and

Rh type and performs a screen for unexpected red cell antibodies, without completing the crossmatch procedure. Because the majority of pretransfusion testing has been performed, compatible blood can be provided rapidly in urgent situations.[3] When clinically significant red cell antibodies are detected in the antibody screen, a crossmatch is performed on units of blood lacking the corresponding antigen(s) in order to ensure rapid availability of compatible blood. Delays may occur in patients who are to undergo surgery on the same day (frequently the same morning) they are admitted to the hospital, because the blood bank may not have sufficient time to identify the antibody. To prevent this occurrence, patients should have blood specimens for compatibility testing drawn prior to the need for blood. For patients with a reliable history of no transfusion or pregnancy within the preceeding 3 months, the 72-hour limit on blood specimen age may be safely extended, eg, up to 14 days. Patients with positive antibody screens and/or special blood requirements may experience delay.

Development and acceptance of MSBOS and type-and-screen programs for elective surgery require a close working relationship among the transfusion, surgery, and anesthesiology services. They require the approval of the transfusion committee of the medical staff or its equivalent.

Alternatives to Allogeneic Blood Transfusion

Every reasonable effort should be made to transfuse blood judiciously. Strategies employed to limit allogeneic blood transfusion may include the use of hematopoietic growth factors, pharmacologic agents to support hemostasis, volume expanders, autologous blood donation (pre-, intra-, and/or postoperatively), and in the near future, artificial oxygen therapeutics (red cell substitutes). Some persons who refuse blood from donors due to religious or other beliefs may accept alternatives to allogeneic blood transfusion.

Preoperative Autologous Blood Collection

Autologous blood transfusion is the process of collection, storage, and reinfusion of a patient's own blood. All patients undergoing elective surgical procedures for which blood replacement is anticipated should be considered as candidates for preoperative blood donation as part of an integrated effort to limit blood transfusion.[4] Advantages include the elimination of the risks of 1) infectious disease transmission; 2) alloimmunization to red cell, platelet, and leukocyte antigens; and 3) immune hemolytic, febrile, allergic, or graft-vs-host reactions. Risks of fluid overload, misidentification leading to ABO-incompatible transfusion, and bacterial contamination, however, are not avoided by autologous transfusion; hence, the indications for autologous blood transfusion should be similar to those for allogeneic transfusion. Preoperative autologous blood donation can provide a source of blood for persons who have either rare blood types or antibodies that make it difficult to find compatible blood.

Participants should be familiar with every aspect of a preoperative autologous blood collection program, such as which blood components are to be collected and stored. Patients must also understand that involvement in such a program does not guarantee transfusion exclusively with their own blood, because unexpected blood loss or inability to collect the desired number of units may occur. Unlike volunteer allogeneic blood donation, no permanent deferral criteria (general information or history) exist for "autologous use only" blood collection. Because there are no specific requirements as to age, both elderly patients and children younger than 17 years of age can participate. For patients weighing less than 110 pounds, it may be necessary to reduce the volume of blood drawn at each donation.[5] Autologous collection during pregnancy seems to be safe, but is usually unnecessary except in selected high-risk obstetric patients.[6]

The medical director of each collection service has the responsibility for overseeing the safety of patient blood donation. Certain guidelines for autologous donors are less stringent than for volunteer donors. The hematocrit should not be less than 33% (hemoglobin 11.0 g/dL) prior to donation. First-time autologous donors who are anemic must be evaluated by a physician to determine the cause of anemia before the first unit can be drawn, because patients are frequently given supplemental iron that can obscure the workup of a patient with unexplained anemia. Because of concurrent medical problems, some patients will not be acceptable candidates for preoperative autologous donation. Criteria for exclusion may vary between facilities. However, the only absolute contraindications to autologous blood donation are current or recent treatment for bacteremia, or the presence of an infectious process that can be associated with bacteremia.[7]

Units for autologous use are usually stored in the liquid state at 1 to 6 C for 35 to 42 days, depending on the anticoagulant-preservative used. If prolonged storage is needed, units can be frozen. A common schedule is to donate 1 unit of blood per week. In adults, the last unit must be donated no later than 72 hours before surgery to avoid hypovolemia at the time of surgery. For patients who require more than 3 units of autologous blood, the administration of recombinant human erythropoietin may facilitate collection of the desired amount. Before transfusion, the ABO and Rh type of the patient and the autologous units should be confirmed.

Orthopedic surgical procedures account for the majority of autologous donor-patients. Autologous donations are also useful in other specialties, including vascular, urologic, and cardiothoracic surgery. A system must be established to manage occasional cancellations or postponements of elective surgery. Unused autologous blood is not used for allogeneic transfusion except in unusual circumstances. Given the potential adverse clinical effects of donation, as well as the anemia, the increased costs associated with autologous transfusion, and the improved safety of allogeneic blood in recent years, the indications for autologous transfusion are being more closely scrutinized.[8,9] The MSBOS or published patient-specific tables may serve as a guide to reduce overcollection.[9]

Acute Normovolemic Hemodilution

Another form of autologous transfusion involves acute normovolemic hemodilution, which refers to the collection of 1 or more units of Whole Blood at the onset of surgery, with reinfusion at the end of the procedure. The volume of blood that is removed and stored in approved plastic blood-collection bags is replaced with crystalloid or colloid solutions. Consequently, blood lost during surgery has a lower hematocrit, thus conserving red cell mass. Furthermore, the reinfused blood provides a source of fresh platelets and clotting factors, which may have been depleted during surgery. This technique is most useful in patients undergoing procedures associated with large-volume blood loss and from whom more than 2 units can be collected.[10] Close patient monitoring is required to guard against fluid overload. The techniques used must ensure that the blood is collected in a sterile manner and properly labeled and stored. Units of blood can be stored at room temperature as long as 8 hours from start of collection or at 1 to 6 C for as long as 24 hours from start of collection, provided 1 to 6 C storage was begun within 8 hours of initiating the collection.[11]

Intraoperative Blood Collection

Intraoperative blood collection is an approach to blood conservation that involves the collection and subsequent reinfusion of blood recovered from the operative site or from an extracorporeal circuit. With this technique, patients can receive their own shed blood, thus minimizing the need for allogeneic blood transfusion. Various types of devices are available for retrieval of blood from the operative site. Such blood may be washed and must be filtered before reinfusion. Blood collected and processed under sterile conditions, and washed with 0.9% saline USP, can be stored as long as 4 hours from the end of collection at room temperature, or as long as 24 hours from the start of collection at 1 to 6 C, provided that refrigeration was begun within 4 hours of initiation of collection.[11] A written protocol describing all procedures involved must be maintained. Blood recovered by intraoperative collection cannot be transfused to other patients. Intraoperative blood collection is generally contraindicated in the presence of systemic infection or malignancy, or with contamination of the surgical field.

Postoperative Blood Collection

Techniques are also available for recovering blood shed postoperatively from surgical drains, chest tubes, or joint cavities. This blood is typically defibrinated and unclottable, and contains high titers of fibrinogen-fibrin degradation products. The collected blood can be processed with or without cell washing, but must be filtered before reinfusion. Blood intended for reinfusion must be given within 6 hours of initiating the collection.[11] The utility of this technique may be limited by the volume and hematocrit of the shed blood.

Directed Blood Donations

Directed blood donations may be made to supply red cells, platelets, plasma, or cryoprecipitate to a specific patient. Medical indications for directed donations include red cells with unusual phenotype, HLA-compatible platelets or granulocytes, and sometimes to supply blood components from a limited pool of donors to a patient who has an infrequent, but predictable requirement. State laws may also mandate that patients be offered the opportunity to procure directed blood donors, and relatives or friends of patients may be highly motivated to donate blood for compassionate reasons or due to a perception of increased safety. There is no evidence to suggest that directed blood donations are safer than volunteer donations and concern has been expressed that directed donors may sometimes be under sufficient social pressure to donate that potential exclusions in the medical history may not be acknowledged by the donor. Directed donations from blood relatives should be irradiated for the prevention of posttransfusion graft-vs-host disease (GVHD).

Urgent and Massive Transfusion

Urgent Transfusion

Urgent transfusion refers to administration of Red Blood Cells (RBCs) before the completion of standard pretransfusion testing, when a delay in transfusion may imperil the patient. Implicit is the understanding that it is necessary to reestablish both oxygen-carrying capacity and intravascular volume. In hypovolemic shock, most authorities recommend immediate volume restoration with crystalloid or colloid solutions. There is controversy regarding the safety of the use of albumin solutions in this setting.[12-14] If volume replacement leads to clinical stabilization, transfusion is less urgent and should await the completion of compatibility testing.

If transfusion is necessary before completion of compatibility testing, group O RBCs should be used. Whenever possible, D-negative RBCs should be used in females of childbearing potential and children to avoid the possibility of sensitization to the D antigen. The patient's physician must sign a statement indicating the nature of the emergency either before or after the uncrossmatched blood is issued. If the patient's screen for unexpected red cell antibodies is negative, the transfusion of uncrossmatched but type-compatible RBCs carries a very low risk of being incompatible.[3] This safety margin is dependent, however, on correct identification of the patient, the pretransfusion blood sample, and the blood components to be infused. Guidelines for conditions under which it is safe to switch the patient to type-specific blood are available.[7] In the near future, administration of artificial oxygen therapeutics may provide a therapeutic bridge to the use of fully compatible blood when emergency transfusion is required.

Massive Transfusion

Massive transfusion is defined as the replacement of one or more blood volumes within 24 hours. A blood volume is estimated as 75 mL/kg or about 5000 mL (10 or more units of Whole Blood) in a 70-kg adult. Patients requiring massive transfusion frequently develop multiple complications related to hypovolemia, tissue ischemia, and acid-base disturbances. Many of these metabolic, coagulation, respiratory, and other complications have been ascribed to the transfusion of stored blood, but are caused principally by tissue damage or hypoperfusion secondary to trauma or hemorrhage.[13,15] Hypothermia may impair hemostasis and should be avoided by warming the patient, the crystalloid solutions administered, and if indicated, the blood.

Massive transfusion may be an indication for the use of Whole Blood. However, Whole Blood may not be available, and RBCs administered with crystalloid or colloid solutions are equally effective in restoring blood volume and oxygen-carrying capacity.[16] The patient's history, vital signs, clinical situation, and hematocrit determine the urgency of red cell support. Plasma and platelet support should be based on the presence or absence of microvascular (not surgical) bleeding and on the results of screening tests of hemostasis [prothrombin time (PT), activated partial thromboplastin time (aPTT), fibrinogen, and platelet count].

Many patients with major hemorrhage who require massive transfusion develop a coagulopathy, but not all develop diffuse microvascular bleeding as a result. This coagulopathy may be characterized by thrombocytopenia, hypofibrinogenemia, and prolongation of the PT and the aPTT. The etiology of this coagulopathy can be multifactorial, and may be caused by consumption of coagulation factors or hemodilution. Patients with severe tissue injury and prolonged hypotension are more likely to develop diffuse microvascular bleeding and require greater hemostatic support.[17] Preestablished formulas to guide component replacement, such as giving 2 units of Fresh Frozen Plasma (FFP) or 6 units of Platelets with every 5 units of RBCs, are not efficacious.[18] Strict reliance on these formulas may provide insufficient support to patients with consumptive coagulopathies and unnecessary transfusion of components to those who do not develop disseminated intravascular coagulation. Through careful monitoring of laboratory tests of hemostasis, the timely and judicious transfusion of Platelets, FFP, or Cryoprecipitated AHF can be reserved for patients with documented deficiencies.

Mild-to-moderate prolongation of the PT or the aPTT does not accurately predict subhemostatic clotting factor levels. Marked prolongations of these tests often reflect factor levels below 20% to 30% (see Overview of Hemostasis), however, and supplemental FFP or Cryoprecipitated AHF may then be indicated.[19] In bleeding patients with thrombocytopenia, platelets should be administered to maintain a platelet count of 50,000/µL. Patients who continue to bleed despite adequate levels of platelets or coagulation factors should be thoroughly re-evaluated and considered for surgical exploration. Close communication between clinicians and the transfusion service director is essential in these cases.

Obstetric Transfusion Practices and Hemolytic Disease of the Newborn

Fetal red cells commonly contain red cell antigens inherited from the father that are lacking in the mother. Fetomaternal hemorrhages occur in nearly all pregnancies; a small percentage of mothers make blood group antibodies against these paternally derived antigens before or after the birth of their offspring. In one study, it was determined that red cell alloimmunization, with development of clinically significant antibodies not associated with transfusions, developed during pregnancy in 0.24% of patients.[20] Maternal IgG antibodies are transported across the placenta and can opsonize fetal red cells, leading to hemolysis of these cells within the fetal spleen. This syndrome, hemolytic disease of the newborn (HDN), can vary in severity from IgG sensitization of fetal red cells without apparent hemolysis to hydropic death in utero caused by severe anemia. IgM antibodies (eg, anti-I, anti-Le[a], anti-P[1]) do not cause HDN because, unlike IgG, they cannot cross the placenta.

The most common cause of clinically significant HDN is antibody to the D antigen. The incidence of Rh hemolytic disease of the newborn is declining, primarily as a result of the use of Rh Immune Globulin (RhIG). The administration of this hyperimmune globulin to pregnant women at risk prevents immunization. Clinically significant HDN due to ABO incompatibility between mother and fetus is rare, even though this serologic situation occurs frequently. Many other blood groups, such as Kell and Duffy, as well as other Rh system antigens, such as c and E, can cause immunization and HDN in both D-positive and D-negative mothers.

The goals of antibody screening in obstetric patients are to identify and monitor those women with blood group antibodies capable of causing HDN and to identify D-negative women who should receive RhIG. Testing at an early prenatal visit should include ABO and Rh typing, as well as an antibody screen designed to detect those red cell antibodies known to cause HDN. If the initial antibody screen is negative, a repeat antibody screen at 28 to 30 weeks of gestation should be considered in D-negative women to detect early D alloimmunization.[21] A 300-μg dose of prophylactic RhIG is administered at this time to all D-negative women.[22] After delivery, all D-negative mothers of Rh-positive infants must also receive a second dose of at least 300 μg of IM RhIG or 120 μg of IV RhIG within 72 hours of birth.[22] A test should be performed to assess whether excessive fetomaternal hemorrhage has occurred, in order to determine if additional RhIG must be administered to prevent D sensitization.[23,24]

If at any time during pregnancy an antibody is identified that is associated with HDN, a titer should be performed and repeated at regular intervals.[23] If a "critical titer" of anti-D of 1:16 or higher is reached, the risk of fetal hydrops after 18 to 20 weeks becomes significant, and further invasive monitoring is indicated. The predictive value of titers for other alloantibodies is uncertain, but an eightfold increase in titer during pregnancy may indicate that the fetal red cells are antigen-positive, and that the fetus is at risk for HDN.[25] Fetal blood type may also be ascertained by determination of the father's red cell phenotype or by genetic amplification testing of fetal DNA derived from amniotic fluid cells, chorionic villi, or maternal plasma.[26] If fetal blood type is determined using genetic testing, cautious interpretation may be necessary, especially if the patient is of African ethnicity. An *RHD* pseudogene has been identified in Rh-negative Africans and African Americans.[27]

Intrauterine Transfusion

Pregnancies complicated by HDN have traditionally been monitored by serial measurement of amniotic fluid bilirubin via amniocentesis in order to assess severity of hemolysis, and by ultrasonography to detect early signs of hydrops. Percutaneous umbilical blood sampling (PUBS) permits antenatal blood typing, precise monitoring of fetal hematocrits, and direct intravascular transfusion (IVT) of the fetus, if necessary. Severely affected fetuses may receive blood either by IVT or intraperitoneal transfusion (IPT) at periodic intervals until assessment of fetal viability indicates sufficient maturity for delivery.[28]

Intrauterine transfusion is generally recommended when the fetal hematocrit falls below 30%, but is rarely feasible before 20 weeks of gestation.[28,29] Blood for transfusion should be serologically compatible with the mother's serum. If the fetal blood type is unknown, group O D-negative RBCs that lack the antigen corresponding to the maternal antibody are used. Freshly donated units of blood, usually less than 1 week old, are preferred in order to maximize survival of the transfused cells. The hematocrit of the red cell component is generally 80% or greater in order to decrease the risk of volume overload in the fetus. The volume transfused is determined according to the gestational age, approximation of fetal blood volume, and the technique to be used for transfusion.[28,29] The mean volume of transfusion using the IVT technique is 50 mL/kg estimated nonhydropic fetal weight, transfused in 10-mL aliquots over 1 to 2 minutes. Transfusions are given when it is estimated that the total circulating hemoglobin concentration has dropped to approximately 10 g/dL, usually every 3 to 4 weeks until the infant is viable.[28,29]

It is recommended that blood for intrauterine transfusion and subsequent exchange transfusion, or any subsequent cellular blood component transfusion, be gamma irradiated [25 Gy (2500 cGy)] to avoid the rare complication of GVHD in the infant. Blood that lacks hemoglobin S should be considered. If the mother is serologically negative for cytomegalovirus (CMV), or her serologic status is unknown, the blood components should be leukocyte-reduced or selected from CMV-seronegative donors, to reduce the risk of CMV disease in the fetus.

Exchange Transfusion

Infants who are severely affected by hemolysis may require exchange transfusion. This technique corrects anemia and removes antibodies and potentially dangerous concentrations of bilirubin. It can be performed in the fetus as well as in the neonate. The blood chosen should be compatible with the mother's serum and ABO-group-compatible with the infant. Blood less than 7 days old is usually used in order to ensure maximum red cell viability and to avoid low pH, decreased red cell 2,3-diphosphoglycerate (2,3-DPG), and high plasma potassium levels. A final hematocrit of 50% to 60% in the component used for exchange is desirable. The use of reconstituted whole blood (ie, RBCs reconstituted with Group AB FFP from a different donor) is most common in exchange transfusion in neonatal nurseries.[29,30]

Blood components should be leukocyte-reduced or selected from CMV-seronegative donors to reduce the risk of CMV disease (see Pediatric Transfusion Practices) in high-risk infants. Blood components for infants who have received intrauterine transfusions should be gamma irradiated (see above). Blood that lacks hemoglobin S should be considered.

Pediatric Transfusion Practices

Transfusion in Neonatal Patients

Two types of anemia develop in premature infants. The first results from the multiple blood sampling that is needed for laboratory monitoring of critically ill preterm infants, while the second develops a few weeks after birth and represents a physiologic decline in hemoglobin concentration. This so-called anemia of prematurity is caused by multiple factors, including inadequate production of and decreased response to endogenous erythropoietin.[31] Although many infants tolerate low hemoglobin levels without clinical difficulties, recombinant erythropoietin may be useful in treating severe anemias of this type.[31,32]

The indications for transfusion in the neonate vary from those in the adult as a result of the infant's physiologic immaturity, small blood volume, and inability to tolerate minimal stress. The decision to transfuse must not be made on the basis of hemoglobin concentration alone, but rather on multiple parameters, including calculated blood loss (generally 5% to 10% of total blood volume) over a given period, expected hemoglobin levels, and clinical status (dyspnea, apnea, pallor, poor weight gain). There are conflicting data, however, on the usefulness of clinical signs (eg, tachycardia, tachypnea, apnea) in an assessment of the need for RBC transfusions in the premature infant.[31] The transfusion of 10 mL/kg of RBCs over a 2- to 3-hour period should raise the hemoglobin concentration by approximately 3 g/dL.

Neonatal transfusion practices vary greatly.[30] Unmodified RBCs are the primary red cell components used by transfusion services to provide small-volume transfusions for neonatal patients. These transfusions generally consist of an aliquot taken from blood units [usually citrate-phosphate-dextrose-adenine (CPDA-1)] less than 7 days old, to minimize excess potassium and maximize 2,3-DPG levels. However, the amount of potassium infused in a small-volume transfusion, even from units stored for 35 to 42 days, is clinically insignificant if the blood is transfused over a 2-hour period at a steady rate.[33,34] If red cells collected in CPDA-1 are not available, red cells in additive solutions can be used safely for small-volume transfusions ($\leq$15 to 20 mL/kg); some transfusion services remove the additive solution by either centrifugation or sedimentation. A sterile connection device may be used to withdraw sequential blood aliquots from an initially fresh (<7 days old) unit of RBCs that is assigned to an infant who is likely to require frequent transfusion.[34] Use of the same unit until its outdate not only provides multiple small-volume transfusions with minimal blood wastage, but also minimizes donor exposure for the neonate.[34,35] This protocol is applicable only to routine transfusions that can be given slowly (2 hours) by infusion pump.

Infants less than 4 months old rarely produce antibodies against blood group antigens; therefore, standards for pretransfusion serologic testing for these patients are different from those for older infants, children, and adults.[7] Before the transfusion is started, ABO and Rh typing, and an antibody screen must be performed. Maternal serum can be used for the latter, because IgG blood group antibodies in infants are passively transferred from mother to infant during gestation. If the initial antibody screen is negative and the RBCs used for transfusion are 1) group O, or ABO-identical or -compatible with both the mother and child, and 2) either the same D-antigen type as the infant or D-negative, then further typing and compatibility testing can be omitted for that admission during the first 4 months of life. If a clinically significant antibody is present, then RBCs lacking the corresponding antigen should be prepared for transfusion for as long as the antibody persists in the infant's serum.

In general, the primary use of FFP is in the treatment of coagulation disorders. Its use is not recommended to treat hypovolemia only. Platelet transfusion practices are variable, including the platelet level at which prophylactic transfusions are given to sick premature infants.[36] The efficacy of granulocyte transfusions in the case of septic and neutropenic neonates is still not fully established.[37]

Transfusion in Older Infants and Children

The decision to transfuse RBCs or other blood components to older infants and children is based on indications similar to those used for adults, taking into consideration the differences in blood volume, the ability to tolerate blood loss, and the normal hemoglobin and hematocrit levels for the age group in question. In certain chronic anemias of childhood, RBC transfusions are utilized to suppress endogenous hemoglobin production. Children with sickle cell disease who are at increased risk for a cerebrovascular accident or who have had major splenic sequestration and are not candidates for splenectomy, may require chronic RBC transfusion to lower the concentration of red cells containing hemoglobin S (Hb S) and to suppress the production of Hb S. Monthly erythrocytapheresis in sickle cell patients who have had a stroke has been effective in minimizing transfusion-related iron overload while preventing recurrence of cerebrovascular accidents. Children with thalassemia syndromes are given routine RBC transfusions to prevent tissue hypoxia and suppress endogenous erythropoiesis in order to support more normal growth and development.[38] To prevent recurrent febrile reactions due to alloimmunization to leukocytes, leukocyte-reduced blood components may be used in patients receiving chronic transfusion. It is prudent to perform extensive red cell phenotyping (including Rh, K, Jk, Fy, Ss) prior to the first transfusion in such patients, because these patients may form complex mixtures of red cell antibodies, and it may be useful to know the phenotype for more efficient antibody identification. In an effort to forestall red cell antibody formation and repeated delayed hemolytic reactions, many facilities use the extended red cell phenotype to administer partially matched red cells.[39]

Cytomegalovirus Infection

Perinatal infection with CMV, although quite variable in its manifestations, can lead to significant morbidity and mortality. This infection can be acquired in utero, during the delivery process, or after birth through breastfeeding, contact with other individuals, or via transfusion. Premature infants born to mothers who are CMV-negative or of unknown serologic status, and who weigh less than 1200 g at birth, have an increased risk of symptomatic transfusion-transmitted CMV. Accordingly, for these or other high-risk patients, it is prudent to transfuse cellular blood components that have been leukocyte-reduced or selected from CMV-negative donors to reduce the risk of CMV transmission.[40] If leukocyte-reduced blood components are used, they must contain <5 × 10^6 leukocytes per final component transfused and be prepared in the laboratory environment where quality can be controlled.

Graft-vs-Host Disease

Posttransfusion GVHD has been reported in pediatric patients with congenital defects in cellular immunity, in infants who have received intrauterine transfusion with or without subsequent exchange transfusion, in children who are immunosuppressed as a result of chemotherapy or irradiation for various malignancies, and rarely, in term infants. Gamma irradiation of cellular blood components is effective in preventing GVHD. Directed donor blood from blood relatives and HLA-matched platelets should be irradiated because of the possibility that the transfusion may cause GVHD.

Neonatal Thrombocytopenia

Neonatal thrombocytopenia may be caused by transmission of maternal antibodies that are reactive with the infant's platelets. This occurs as a result of sensitization of the mother to the infant's platelet antigens, particularly HPA-1a (Pl^{A1}) in a manner analogous to hemolytic disease of the newborn, or rarely, as a result of maternal idiopathic thrombocytopenic purpura (ITP). While maternal ITP typically runs a benign course in the infant, neonatal alloimmune thrombocytopenia frequently affects the firstborn infant and can cause serious intracranial hemorrhage, even before delivery.[42] This condition may be treated in utero by administration of intravenous gammaglobulin (IVIG) to the mother or by direct intravascular transfusion with compatible platelets (washed or plasma-reduced maternal platelets).[42] It may also be necessary to transfuse platelets postpartum. Antigen-negative platelets may sometimes be required.[42]

Management of Platelet Alloimmunization

Patients who repeatedly fail to achieve a therapeutic increment in platelet count following platelet transfusion are said to be refractory. The posttransfusion platelet count increment can be calculated and used to confirm the development of the refractory state (see Platelets). The onset of refractoriness may be associated with difficulty in controlling clinical bleeding and with repeated febrile reactions to platelet transfusion. In most patients, refractoriness results from nonimmune causes, but refractoriness is also frequently due to the development of alloantibodies directed against foreign HLA and/or platelet-specific antigens.

The most common alloantibodies that lead to platelet refractoriness are directed against Class I antigens in the HLA system. These antigens are expressed on many different cell types, including platelets and lymphocytes. HLA antibodies develop after exposure to foreign HLA antigens, as may occur during pregnancy or after transfusions of cellular blood components. Less commonly, patients become refractory due to platelet-specific (non-HLA) antibodies, to ABO incompatibility, or to drug-induced antibodies. The possibility of ITP or posttransfusion purpura (PTP) should also be considered. The diagnosis of allo-immunization is supported by a positive test for antibodies to HLA antigens or by a positive platelet crossmatch.

Effective therapies for alloimmunized patients with severe thrombocytopenia are limited. Platelet transfusions from random donors are nearly always ineffective, but the use of platelets from family members or HLA-matched donors often restores platelet responsiveness.[43] The extensive polymorphism of the HLA system, however, precludes the procurement of sufficient HLA-identical donors to satisfy the needs of most refractory patients. The transfusion of platelets from partially or selectively HLA-matched donors may be successful if the match is close enough.[44,45] Identifying the specificity of the HLA antibody (analogous to red cell antibody identification) may permit a wider choice of donors with known HLA types. Platelet crossmatching, in which patient serum is tested with a panel of single-donor platelets, the least reactive of which is selected for transfusion, has also been successful.[46,47] Platelet crossmatching has the advantage of detecting both HLA and platelet-specific antibodies, but this technique is not available in all blood centers.

In some cases, even the use of well-matched platelets does not result in adequate posttransfusion increments. This may be due to the presence of complicating nonimmune factors or to platelet ABO incompatibility.[48,49] Other methods of circumventing allo-immunization, such as the use of high-dose IVIG, plasmapheresis, splenectomy, or epsilon-aminocaproic acid, have met with marginal success.

Because treatment of the refractory patient remains problematic, the prevention of primary HLA immunization has become a major focus of investigation. The prophylactic use of HLA-identical platelets should prevent alloimmunization, but is not feasible.

Evidence indicates that platelets themselves are not highly immunogenic, and that passenger leukocytes in the transfusion product are responsible for induction of platelet antibodies. A randomized multicenter trial demonstrated that the prophylactic use of platelets and red cells that underwent leukocyte reduction through the use of third-generation filters decreased the rate of alloimmunization and refractoriness in multitransfused patients with acute leukemia, including women who had previously been pregnant.[50] No advantage was found for the use of Platelets Pheresis Leukocytes Reduced vs pooled Platelets Leukocytes Reduced. Leukocyte reduction of cellular blood components is thus indicated in all patients with acute leukemia. It is not clear if exclusive use of leukocyte-reduced blood components will prevent HLA alloimmunization in patients with other hematologic malignancies. The irradiation of platelets with ultraviolet-B light also prevented alloimmunization; however, this technique is not readily available.[50]

Solid Organ Transplantation

The transplantation of solid organs, such as kidney, heart, lung, small bowel, and liver, poses different challenges for transfusion therapy. The transplant procedure and perioperative period may be associated with substantial bleeding. Solid organ transplant surgeries, except kidney, typically require both RBC and plasma transfusion.

Median blood component requirements in adult liver transplantation are typically 10 to 12 units each of RBCs, Plasma, and Platelets, and 0 to 5 units of Cryoprecipitated AHF.[51] Liver transplant patients often have complex preoperative coagulopathies that may be compounded during the anhepatic phase of surgery to yield profound hemostatic derangements. In severe cases, a single liver transplant recipient may tax the available blood supply of an entire community. Normal hemostasis gradually resumes once the transplanted liver begins to function.

ABO compatibility is a primary concern in solid organ transplants. Transplantation across major ABO barriers (eg, A donor to O recipient) will often result in rapid rejection, especially of hearts and kidneys.[52] Minor ABO incompatibility is not as dangerous, but can be associated with significant hemolytic anemia caused by ABO (or other red cell) antibody production by passenger graft lymphocytes.

HLA alloimmunization in solid organ transplantation can also result in rejection of the engrafted organ due to preexisting HLA antibodies. This may have importance in kidney, heart, lung, and perhaps liver transplants.[52] Graft survival is enhanced in the setting of highly HLA-matched donor-recipient combinations.[53] In renal transplantation, lymphocytotoxic crossmatching between patient serum and donor lymphocytes is performed routinely when a donor kidney becomes available and may predict success. HLA-alloimmunized liver transplant recipients generally have a marked increase in blood component requirements during surgery.[54]

The transfusion of cellular blood components before kidney transplantation is known to have a favorable effect on graft survival, but the mechanism of the effect is poorly understood.[55] The advent of newer immunosuppressive agents has nearly eliminated the clinical benefit of preoperative transfusions, which are no longer routinely performed.[56]

GVHD is not commonly seen after solid organ transplantation. It has been reported in a few cases, however, having been caused by the passive transfer of immunocompetent lymphocytes in donor organs.[57] Because cases of transfusion-associated GVHD have occurred only rarely in this setting, the use of irradiated blood components for solid organ recipients is not routinely required.

Administration of Blood

The most common cause of fatal hemolytic transfusion reactions is the misidentification of either the blood unit or the recipient. Among the steps necessary for safe transfusion, the positive identification of the patient and the blood sample is of critical importance. After sample collection, identification systems inside and outside the blood bank must be in place to ensure that technical and clerical errors are not made.

At the time of transfusion, the blood component unit with the compatibility tag attached (this tag should not be removed) must be compared with the patient's identification bracelet. No discrepancies in spelling or identification numbers should exist. The patient should remain under direct observation for 5 to 10 minutes after the infusion begins and must be assessed periodically until an appropriate time after the transfusion is completed.[7]

Blood Warming

Transfusion of cold blood at rates exceeding 100 mL/minute has been associated with a higher rate of cardiac arrest when compared with rates in a control group receiving warm blood.[58] However, patients receiving blood at a slow rate do not routinely require warmed blood.

Blood warmers are of two types: 1) a coil of plastic tubing placed in a temperature-monitored waterbath, and 2) electrically heated plates in contact with a flat plastic blood bag. Automatic warming devices must have a visible thermometer and should have an audible warning system. Warming the whole unit of blood by immersion in hot water or by the use of microwave blood warmers is contraindicated because hemolysis can result from overheating.[59]

The use of blood warmers is generally restricted to adult patients receiving rapid and multiple transfusions (rate over 50 mL/kg/hour), exchange transfusions in infants, children receiving blood in volumes in excess of 15 mL/kg/hour, and patients with severe cold autoimmune hemolytic anemia.

Time Limits for Infusing Blood Components

A unit of blood should not be kept at room temperature for more than a short time due to the risk of bacterial growth. Blood should be infused within 4 hours. If that time is likely to be exceeded, the unit should be divided into aliquots, and portions should be kept in the blood bank refrigerator until required. A unit of blood that has been allowed to warm above 10 C, but is not used, cannot be reissued by the transfusion service. Blood must never be stored in unmonitored refrigerators.

Concomitant Use of Intravenous Solutions

Only normal saline (0.9% USP) may be administered with blood components. Other solutions may be hypotonic (eg, 5% dextrose in water) and cause hemolysis in vitro, or may contain additives such as calcium (Ringer's lactate) that can initiate in-vitro coagulation in citrated blood.[60] To increase infusion rate and decrease viscosity, RBCs may be diluted with normal saline (0.9% USP). Medications should never be added to a unit of blood or infused with blood, for several reasons. Some drugs may cause hemolysis due to their excessively high pH. Furthermore, if medication is added to blood and the transfusion is discontinued for any reason, the dose of infused medication may not be known. Finally, it would be difficult to determine whether any adverse transfusion reactions were due to the blood or to the drug it contained.

Filters

All blood components must be administered through a filter in order to remove blood clots and other debris. Standard blood filters, with a pore size between 150 and 280 microns, trap large aggregates and clots. Microaggregate blood filters with 20- to 40-micron pores can remove microaggregate debris, and are frequently employed when blood is recirculated in cardiac bypass devices. They are not indicated for routine blood transfusions and do not accomplish leukocyte reduction. Third-generation blood filters are available for provision of leukocyte-reduced cellular blood components (see Red Blood Cells Leukocytes Reduced). Disadvantages of both microaggregate and leukocyte reduction filters include the potential to become clogged and resistance to rapid blood delivery. These problems may be circumvented by using components that have been leukocyte-reduced in the laboratory prior to issue.

Infusion Devices

Several electronic infusion devices ("blood pumps") are available. These machines are designed to deliver parenteral fluids, including blood components, at flow rates as low as 1 mL/hour. The pump mechanisms vary with different manufacturers and include syringe-type pumping systems, peristaltic roller devices, and electromechanical pumps that operate on a positive volumetric displacement principle.

Some systems require manufacturer-supplied pump cassettes, while others can be used with standard intravenous administration set tubing. Although most pump systems do not induce mechanical hemolysis when used with Whole Blood, gross hemolysis can result when some models are used to administer RBCs. Manufacturer's insert should be consulted for approval for use with blood components. Rapid infusion devices are available that can infuse blood at a rate as high as 2 L/minute.[61]

References

1. Friedman BA. An analysis of surgical blood use in United States hospitals with applications to the maximum surgical blood order schedule. Transfusion 1979;19:268-78.

2. Popovsky MA, Triulzi DJ. The effects of managed care on transfusion medicine. Transfus Med Rev 1997;11:195-9.

3. Oberman HA, Barnes BA, Friedman BA. The risk of abbreviating the major crossmatch in urgent or massive transfusion. Transfusion 1978;18:137-41.

4. Goodnough LT, Brecher ME. Autologous blood transfusion. Intern Med 1998;37(3):238-45.

5. Silvergleid AJ. Safety and effectiveness of predeposit autologous transfusions in preteen and adolescent children. JAMA 1987;257:3403-4.

6. Pepkowitz SH. Autologous blood donation and obstetric transfusion practice. In: Sacher RA, Brecher ME, eds. Obstetric transfusion practice. Bethesda, MD: American Association of Blood Banks, 1993:77-94.

7. Gorlin JB, ed. Standards for blood banks and transfusion services, 21st ed. Bethesda, MD: American Association of Blood Banks, 2002.

8. Etchason J, Petz L, Keeler E, et al. The cost-effectiveness of preoperative autologous blood donations. N Engl J Med 1995;332:719-24.

9. Brecher ME, Monk T, Goodnough LT. A standardized method for calculating blood loss. Transfusion 1997;37:1070-4.

10. Weiskopf RB. Mathematical analysis of isovolemic hemodilution indicates that it can decrease the need for allogeneic blood transfusion. Transfusion 1995;35:37-41.

11. Santrach PJ, ed. Standards for perioperative autologous blood collection and administration, 1st ed. Bethesda, MD: American Association of Blood Banks, 2001.

12. Cochrane Injuries Group Albumin Reviewers. Human albumin administration in critically ill patients: Systematic review of randomised controlled trials. Br Med J 1998;317:235-40.

13. Collins JA. Massive blood transfusions. Clin Haematol 1976;5:201-22.

14. Moss GS, Gould S. Plasma expanders—an update. Surg Pharmacol 1988;155:425-34.

15. Mannucci PM, Federici AB, Sirchia G. Hemostasis testing during massive blood replacement: A study of 172 cases. Vox Sang 1982;42:113-23.

16. Shackford SR, Virgilio R, Peters RM. Whole blood versus packed-cell transfusions. Ann Surg 1981;193:337-40.

17. Collins JA. Recent developments in the area of massive transfusion. World J Surg 1987;11:75-81.

18. Reed RL, Ciavarella D, Heimbach DM, et al. Prophylactic platelet administration during massive transfusion. Ann Surg 1986;203:40-8.

19. Ciavarella D, Reed RL, Counts RB, et al. Clotting factor levels and the risk of diffuse microvascular bleeding in the massively transfused patient. Br J Haematol 1987;67:365-8.

20. Heddle NM, Klama L, Frassetto R, et al. A retrospective study to determine the risk of red cell alloimmunization

and transfusion during pregnancy. Transfusion 1993;33: 217-20.

21. Hartwell EA. Use of Rh immune globulin: ASCP practice parameter. Am J Clin Pathol 1998;110:281-92.

22. American College of Obstetrics and Gynecology. Prevention of Rh$_o$(D) isoimmunization. ACOG Tech Bull 1984; 79:1-4.

23. Management of isoimmunization in pregnancy: ACOG educational bulletin. Int J Gynecol Obstet 1996;55:183-90.

24. Prevention of hemolytic disease of the newborn due to anti-D. Association Bulletin #98-2. Bethesda, MD: American Association of Blood Banks, 1998.

25. Brecher ME, ed. Technical Manual, 14th ed. Bethesda, MD: American Association of Blood Banks, 2002:497-513.

26. Lo YM, Hjelm NM, Fidler C, et al. Prenatal diagnosis of fetal RhD status by molecular analysis of maternal plasma. N Engl J Med 1998;339:1734-8.

27. Singleton BK, Green CA, Avent ND, et al. The presence of an RHD pseudogene containing a 37 base pair duplication and a nonsense mutation in Africans with the Rh D-negative blood group phenotype. Blood 2000;95:12-8.

28. Bowman J. The management of hemolytic disease in the fetus and newborn. Semin Perinatol 1997;211:39-44.

29. Moise KJ. Management of red cell alloimmunization in pregnancy. In: Sacher RA, Brecher ME, eds. Obstetric transfusion practice. Bethesda, MD: American Association of Blood Banks, 1993:21-47.

30. Hume H, Blanchette V, Strauss RG, Levy GJ. A survey of Canadian neonatal blood transfusion practices. Transfus Sci 1997;18(1):71-80.

31. Shannon KM. Anemia of prematurity: Progress and prospects. Am J Pediatr Hematol Oncol 1990;12:14-20.

32. Carnielli V, Montini G, DaRiol R, et al. Effect of high doses of human recombinant erythropoietin on the need for blood transfusions in preterm infants. J Pediatr 1992; 121:98-102.

33. Luban NLC, Strauss RG, Hume HA. Commentary on the safety of red cells preserved in extended-storage media for neonatal transfusions. Transfusion 1991;31:229-35.

34. Lui EA, Mannino FL, Lane TA. A prospective, randomized trial of the safety and efficacy of a limited donor exposure transfusion program in premature neonates. J Pediatr 1994;125:92-6.

35. Wang-Rodriquez J, Mannino FL, Liu E, Lane TA. A novel strategy to limit blood donor exposure and blood wastage in multiply transfused premature infants. Transfusion 1996;36:64-70.

36. Strauss RG, Blanchette VS, Hume H, et al. National acceptability of American Association of Blood Banks Pediatric Hemotherapy Committee guidelines for auditing pediatric transfusion practices. Transfusion 1993;33:168-71.

37. Sweetman RW, Cairo MS. Blood component and immunotherapy in neonatal sepsis. Transfus Med Rev 1995;9(3):251-9.

38. DePalma L, Ness PM, Luban NLC. Red blood cell transfusion. In: Luban NLC, ed. Transfusion therapy in infants and children. Baltimore, MD: The Johns Hopkins University Press, 1991:1-30.

39. Vichinsky EP, Earles A, Johnson RA, et al. Alloimmunization in sickle cell anemia and transfusion of racially unmatched blood. N Engl J Med 1990;322:1617-21.

40. Sayers MH, Anderson KC, Goodnough LT, et al. Reducing the risk for transfusion-transmitted cytomegalovirus infection. Ann Intern Med 1992;116:55-62.

41. Popovsky MA. Quality of blood components filtered before storage and at the bedside: Implications for transfusion practice. Transfusion 1996;36:470-4.

42. Kaplan C, Forestier F, Daffos F, et al. Management of fetal and neonatal alloimmune thrombocytopenia. Transfus Med Rev 1996;10:233-40.

43. Yankee RA, Grumet FC, Rogentine GN. Platelet transfusion therapy: The selection of compatible platelet donors for refractory patients by lymphocyte HLA typing. N Engl J Med 1969;281:1208-12.

44. Duquesnoy RJ, Filip DJ, Rodey, GE, et al. Successful transfusion of platelets mismatched for HLA antigens to

alloimmunized thrombocytopenic patients. Am J Hematol 1977;2:219-26.

45. Dahlke MB, Weiss KL. Platelet transfusion from donors mismatched for crossreactive HLA antigens. Transfusion 1984;24:299-302.

46. O'Connell BA, Lee ES, Rothko K, Schiffer CA. Selection of histocompatible apheresis platelet donors by cross-matching random platelet concentrates. Blood 1992;79: 527-31.

47. Moroff G, Garratty G, Heal JM, et al. Selection of platelets for refractory patients by HLA matching and prospective crossmatching. Transfusion 1992;32(7):633-40.

48. Friedberg RC, Donnelly SF, Boyd JC, et al. Clinical and blood bank factors in the management of platelet refracto-riness and alloimmunization. Blood 1993;81:3482-34.

49. Lee EJ, Schiffer CA. ABO compatibility can influence the results of platelet transfusion. Transfusion 1989;29:384-7.

50. Leukocyte reduction and ultraviolet B irradiation of plate-lets to prevent alloimmunization and refractoriness to platelet transfusions. The Trial to Reduce Alloimmuni-zation to Platelets Study. N Engl J Med 1997;337(26): 1861-9.

51. Triulzi DJ. Transfusion support in solid-organ transplanta-tion. In: Reid ME, Nance SJ, eds. Red cell transfusion: A practical guide. Totowa, NJ: Humana Press Inc, 1998: 105-19.

52. Ramsey G, Sherman LA. Transfusion therapy in solid or-gan transplantation. Hematol Oncol Clin North Am 1994; 8:1117-29.

53. Opelz G, Wujciak T. The influence of HLA compatibility on graft survival after heart transplantation. N Engl J Med 1994;330:816-20.

54. Takaya S, Bronsther O, Iwaki Y, et al. The adverse impact on liver transplantation of using positive cytotoxic cross-match donors. Transplantation 1992;53:400-3.

55. Opelz G, Sengar DPS, Mickey MR, et al. Effect of blood transfusion on subsequent kidney transplants. Transplant Proc 1973;5:253-59.

56. Opelz G. Improved kidney graft survival in nontransfused recipients. Transplant Proc 1987;19:149-52.
57. Triulzi DJ, Nalesnik MA. Microchimerism, GVHD, and tolerance in solid organ transplantation. Transfusion 2001; 41:419-26.
58. Boyan CP, Howland WS. Cardiac arrest and temperature of bank blood. JAMA 1963;183:58-60.
59. Arens JF, Leonard GL. Danger of overwarming blood by microwave. JAMA 1971;218:1045-6.
60. Ryden SE, Oberman HA. Compatibility of common intravenous solutions with CPD blood. Transfusion 1975;15: 250-5.
61. Sassano JJ. The rapid infusion system. In: Winter PM, Kang YG, eds. Hepatic transplantation: Anesthetic and perioperative management. New York: Praeger, 1986: 120-34.

HEMOSTATIC DISORDERS

Overview of Hemostasis

Hemostasis refers to the physiologic mechanisms that result in the control of bleeding. Normal hemostasis may be viewed as occurring in three stages, although it should be kept in mind that these overlap. Primary hemostasis involves: blood vessels (particularly the endothelial layer) and cellular blood elements (particularly platelets) and formation of the platelet plug. The second stage of hemostasis involves plasma procoagulant proteins (clotting or coagulation factors) and formation of a stable fibrin clot. In the third stage, repair of vascular damage results in a return to the normal state. Two control processes, the fibrinolytic system and inhibitory (or anticoagulant) proteins are important in limiting clot formation. Pathologic bleeding or thrombosis may result from derangements in any of these processes.

Blood Vessels

The normal endothelium is maintained as a thromboresistant surface by a variety of mechanisms, including the production of the antiplatelet prostaglandin prostacyclin. Following injury, the blood vessel constricts, limiting blood flow. Exposure of subendothelial structures leads to adhesion and activation of platelets and stimulates activation of the procoagulant elements of the system. Platelets adhere to subendothelium in seconds, followed within minutes by fibrin formation and a stable platelet-fibrin clot.

Hereditary blood vessel disorders associated with a bleeding diathesis include rare disorders of vessel connective tissue structures, such as Ehlers-Danlos and Marfan syndromes. Vascular malformations, which can cause recurrent bleeding, include telangiectasia (Rendu-Osler-Weber syndrome), angiodysplasia, and giant hemangioma.

Acquired blood vessel disorders include trauma, scurvy, and vasculitis. Treatment is directed to the underlying problem.

Postoperative anatomic bleeding due to inadequate surgical hemostasis may be difficult to diagnose, particularly in patients with abnormalities of platelets or coagulation factors. In general, bleeding from one site suggests anatomical bleeding, while small-vessel bleeding from multiple sites (wound edges, IV sites, endotracheal tube) suggests abnormal hemostasis.

Platelets

Platelets are anuclear cells that form a cohesive plug at the site of vessel injury.

Thrombocytopenia and platelet function defects are both causes of abnormal hemostasis. Platelet function is routinely assessed by two screening tests: the platelet count and platelet function assays. In patients who are actively bleeding or who are about to undergo major invasive procedures, platelet transfusions are often indicated for counts less than 50,000/μL.[1,2] Higher counts may be required for procedures where any increased bleeding would be problematic, such as neurologic or ophthalmologic surgery. In nonbleeding patients, prophylactic platelet transfusions are indicated at counts below 5000 to 10,000/μL.[3,4] With clinical factors such as fever, sepsis, splenomegaly, renal failure or drugs (eg, amphotericin), a higher threshold (ie, 20,000/μL) may be needed.[5,6]

Studies have cast doubt on the value of the bleeding time in predicting surgical bleeding.[7,8] Bleeding time may be prolonged at platelet counts below 100,000/μL. Bleeding times are most useful as an aid in evaluation of an apparent hemostatic defect.

The closure time is an in-vitro bleeding time, performed by platelet function analyzer 100 (PFA 100). Closure time refers to the time required for a platelet aggregate to occlude the aperture of a collagen-coated membrane.[9,10] It is sensitive to platelet aggregation abnormalities (aspirin effect, Glanzmann's thrombasthenia) and von Willebrand disease (vWD). Many institutions have replaced bleeding time with closure time. Neither of these tests is superior to a detailed bleeding history.

Abnormal bleeding or closure time with an adequate platelet count should be followed by platelet aggregation study and/or measurements of von Willebrand factor (vWF).

Platelets serve an important role in the coagulation system as well. Coagulation proteins and Ca^{++} are stored within platelet granules and coagulation factors assemble on the phospholipid surface of activated platelets. Glycoprotein (GP)IIb-IIIa inhibitors (abciximab, eptifibatide, tirofiban) are newly licensed drugs that inhibit platelet aggregation, namely the binding of fibrinogen or vWF to the GPIIb-IIIa receptor. These drugs significantly reduce thrombotic complications in patients with acute coronary syndromes undergoing percutaneous coronary intervention.[11] They inhibit thrombin generation and platelet procoagulant activity and prolong the activated clotting time. Patients who develop bleeding after having received GPIIb-IIIa inhibitors may require repeated platelet transfusion to counteract the effect of the drug. Thrombocytopenia is an infrequent complication of GPIIb-IIIa inhibitor therapy, seen in less than 1.0 % of cases.[12] Discontinuation of the GPIIb-IIIa inhibitor and, in severe cases, platelet transfusion is recommended.

Coagulation Proteins

The coagulation mechanism consists of a closely regulated series of reactions culminating in the formation of an insoluble protein gel called fibrin. The initial platelet plug, which is woven with fibrin strands, stabilizes the clot. The system consists of procoagulant serine proteases that circulate as zymogens (Factors II, VII, IX, X, XI, XII), nonenzymatic cofactors (Factors V, VIII), fibrinogen, the substrate for the fibrin gel, and a fibrin-stabilizing enzyme, Factor XIII.

In vivo, the exposure of tissue factor (TF) to blood is the key step in the initiation of coagulation.[13] TF is abundantly present in the subendothelium and it triggers the coagulation system at the site of injury by binding to circulating Factor VIIa. The Factor VIIa-TF complex converts Factor X to its active form either directly or indirectly. The Factor VIIa-TF complex indirectly activates Factor X by activating Factor IX. Factor IX requires Factor VIIIa as a co-factor for activity. Prothrombin is activated by the prothrombinase complex, which consists of phospholipid bound Factors Xa and Va. Thrombin dissociates from the membrane surface and converts fibrinogen to fibrin. Factor XIIIa stabilizes the clot by covalent cross-linking of fibrin. Thrombin amplifies the coagulation system by feedback activation of Factors XI, VIII, and V. This positive feedback sustains coagulation after the Factor VIIa-TF process is inhibited by TF pathway inhibitor. This could explain why hemophiliacs bleed despite normal levels of Factor VII.

In vitro, coagulation can be initiated by another protease/co-factor system, the so-called contact factor system. Deficiencies of these proteins (Factor XII, prekallikrein, and kininogen) will prolong screening tests of hemostasis usually without giving rise to a bleeding diathesis in vivo.

Screening tests of coagulation include the prothrombin time (PT; evaluates the extrinsic pathway that includes Factors VII, X, V, and II and fibrinogen), the activated partial thromboplastin time (aPTT; evaluates the intrinsic pathway that includes prekallikrein and kininogen, Factors XII, XI, IX, VIII, X, V, and II and fibrinogen), the thrombin time (TT; evaluates the fibrinogen-to-fibrin conversion step and is sensitive to the effect of heparin), and a quantitative fibrinogen assay. Acquired mild-to-moderate prolongations of the PT, aPTT, and TT due to liver disease or dilution are not often associated with significant decreases in coagulation factor levels or with an increased bleeding risk.[14] However, in congenital hemostatic disorders, mild abnormalities in the PT or the aPTT may be clinically significant. The therapeutic levels of these factors required for hemostasis and the indications for factor replacement depend upon the patients clinical status. In general, factor levels above 25% to 35% and fibrinogen levels above 100 mg/dL are sufficient to prevent major hemorrhage.

Both congenital and acquired disorders of coagulation occur. Common congenital disorders include von Willebrand disease and the hemophilias, while common acquired disorders include liver disease and consumptive coagulopathy. Whenever possible, patients with disorders of coagulation determined by history or screening tests should be treated in consultation with a hematologist.

Natural Anticoagulant Systems and Fibrinolysis

The processes by which procoagulant activities are limited to the site of injury, and the repair initiated, are important regulators of normal hemostasis. Two main processes are involved: the natural anticoagulant systems, which consists primarily of circulating and endothelial-based protease inhibitors, and the fibrinolytic system, which is responsible for the proteolytic dissolution of the fibrin clot.

Blood fluidity depends largely on the integrity of two natural anticoagulant systems. In the first system, antithrombin inhibits thrombin and other free coagulation factors to protect the circulation from liberated enzymes. Antithrombin is a weak inhibitor by itself, but heparin and heparin-like molecules markedly augment its activity. In the second system, thrombin binds to thrombomodulin on endothelial cells and activates protein C. Activated protein C, in the presence of protein S, inactivates Factors Va and VIIIa. A mutation in Factor V (Factor V Leiden) results in resistance to the anticoagulant action of activated protein C.[15]

Fibrinolysis is accomplished by the enzyme plasmin, which is formed by the action of endothelium-based activators upon its circulating zymogen, plasminogen. Plasminogen activator (tissue type or urokinase type) converts plasminogen to plasmin. Plasmin binds to the newly formed fibrin and breaks it down to soluble degradation products, leading to clot lysis. Unbound plasmin can degrade fibrinogen, Factor V, and Factor VIII. In-vivo regulation of plasmin activity occurs at two levels: 1) plasminogen activator inhibitor (PAI) blocks the activation of plasminogen by the plasminogen acivators; and 2) alpha$_2$-antiplasmin inhibits plasmin. An increased level of plasminogen activator or a deficiency of PAI or deficiency of alpha$_2$-antiplasmin may cause a bleeding tendency by increasing the plasmin level.

Conversely, an increased level of PAI, resistance of fibrin to the normal action of plasmin in thrombotic dysfibrinogenemias, dysfunctional or decreased plasminogen, and decreased activation of plasminogen have all been described and are associated with increased thrombotic risk. The link between fibrinolysis and coagulation is the newly discovered thrombin activatable fibrinolysis inhibitor (TAFI). As its name indicates, TAFI is activated by thrombin and it reduces the efficiency of clot lysis by plasmin. Elevated TAFI levels were found to be associated with a mild risk for venous thrombosis.[16]

The laboratory hallmark of an activated fibrinolytic system is the detection of free plasmin in the blood. However, no direct assay is available; instead, a shortened (<60 min) euglobulin clot lysis time indicates a fibrinolytic state. Several other test results may also point to activated fibrinolysis, such as a drop in the plasma fibrinogen level or an elevation of TT, aPTT, or the fibrin(ogen) degradation products. An elevation of these degradation products can inhibit fibrin formation and impair platelet function. The thromboelastogram (TEG) shows early decrease in clot strength with accelerated fibrinolysis.[17]

Severe liver disease and hepatic surgery (resection or transplantation) are the most common causes of primary fibrinolysis.

Platelet Disorders

Many conditions can result in thrombocytopenia. When it results from marrow suppression (radiation, chemotherapy, nutritional deficiency, or toxic drugs), platelet transfusions are usually successful in elevating the platelet count and lowering bleeding risk. In contrast, accelerated destruction of peripheral blood platelets, (consumptive or immune disorders) is more difficult to treat with transfusions because the transfused platelets are also rapidly destroyed. Platelet transfusions are generally not indicated in autoimmune or adult alloimmune thrombocytopenia because the survival of the transfused platelets is very brief,[1] although exceptions occur.[18] Platelet transfusion should be avoided in patients with thrombotic thrombocytopenic purpura or heparin-induced thrombocytopenia to avoid exacerbation of thrombosis.[19] Patients who have been repeatedly transfused or pregnant may also develop antibodies to HLA antigens present on the platelet surface and become refractory to platelets. Frequently these patients will respond to transfusions of platelets that are crossmatch negative or matched for their HLA type. The prophylactic use of leukocyte-reduced blood components reduces the rate of alloimmunization and refractoriness to platelet transfusions in patients with acute leukemia.[20]

Platelet function defects may be congenital or acquired. Congenital disorders include abnormalities of platelet granules or membrane receptors. Acquired disorders are most often caused by drugs, especially aspirin, nonsteroidal anti-inflammatory agents, and GPIIb/IIIa inhibitors. Patients with uremia and those undergoing procedures using extracorporeal circulation often have platelet function defects. Platelet transfusion can be used to treat selected platelet function defects. The hemostatic defect seen with uremia will not respond to platelet transfusion alone.

Desmopressin (DDAVP) has been reported to be effective in treating bleeding in uremia and in treating congenital platelet function abnormalities. DDAVP releases Factor VIII and vWF from endothelial cells and other storage sites. The mechanism of action in the improvement of platelet function is unclear, but it may relate to elevated levels of the adhesive protein, vWF. Treatment of bleeding in uremic patients without thrombocytopenia includes dialysis; maintenance of the hematocrit >30%[21] administration of DDAVP and conjugated estrogens.

Congenital Bleeding Disorders

von Willebrand Disease

The most common hereditary bleeding disorder is von Willebrand disease.[22] It may result from quantitative or qualitative abnormalities of von Willebrand factor, a large multimeric molecule. It binds, carries, and protects Factor VIII in plasma. Platelet adhesion to subendothelial tissue requires vWF; therefore, platelet plug formation is deficient in patients with vWD. Diminished Factor VIII levels are seen in patients with vWD secondary to low vWF levels. Von Willebrand disease is manifested as a platelet function defect characterized most commonly by mucosal bleeding, but deep tissue bleeding can occur in severe cases. The diagnosis is confirmed by specific assays for vWF and Factor VIII. Most forms of mild or moderate vWD can be treated with DDAVP.[23] DDAVP is contraindicated in individuals with the rare type 2b variant and not useful in type 3 variant, where vWF is absent. It is administered as intravenous and subcutaneous injection or as concentrated nasal spray (Stimate). DDAVP is usually given in doses of 0.3 µg/kg intravenously over 20 minutes. The majority of patients experience a two- to threefold increase of vWF 30 to 60 minutes after infusion and the effect persists for about 6 hours.[24] Tachyphylaxis may develop with repeated doses; therefore, DDAVP is usually not effective after 3 to 4 consecutive daily doses. Mild and transient side effects include headache and facial flushing. To prevent hyponatremia and water retention due to the antidiuretic effect of DDAVP, patients should restrict fluid intake for 24 hours after administration. It should be used with caution in elderly individuals with cardiovascular disease and small children weighing <20 kg.

Patients who are unresponsive to DDAVP or have type 2b and type 3 variants require exogenous vWF-containing concentrates. Virus-inactivated products (Humate-P, Alphanate, Koate) are recommended.[23] Concerns over transfusion-transmitted disease have made treatment with FFP and Cryoprecipitated AHF less desirable. Factor VIII concentrates prepared by monoclonal or recombinant technology are devoid of vWF.

Hemophilia A—Factor VIII Deficiency

Hemophilia A is an X-linked congenital bleeding disorder, caused by Factor VIII deficiency. Both gene deletions and point mutations have been described.[25] The vWF levels are normal. Patients with Factor VIII levels above 5% are considered mild hemophiliacs, and significant trauma usually precedes bleeding episodes.

Moderate hemophiliacs have Factor VIII levels of 1% to 5% and can have excessive bleeding with minimal trauma or after surgery. Severe hemophiliacs (Factor VIII levels less than 1%) are at risk for spontaneous hemorrhage.

Unlike platelet-related bleeding, hemophilic bleeding manifests several hours after the causative trauma and occurs most frequently in deep structures, such as joints and muscles. Bleeding may occur anywhere, however, including in the brain and the gastrointestinal tract.

Mild or moderate hemophilia A can be treated with DDAVP, whereas severe disease requires the infusion of Factor VIII concentrates. Virus-inactivated and recombinant Factor VIII concentrates are the products of choice. First- and second-generation recombinant Factor VIII concentrates are now available (see Factor VIII Concentrate). Monitoring B-domain-deleted recombinant Factor VIII therapy requires either a chromogenic assay or a modified one-stage aPTT-based assay calibrated to a specific standard.[26]

Hemophilia B—Factor IX Deficiency

The clinical manifestations of Factor IX deficiency are identical to those of Factor VIII deficiency. Factor IX is replaced with Factor IX concentrates, which are predominantly produced from recombinant sources (see Chapter 2). DDAVP and Cryoprecipitated AHF are *not* effective in the treatment of individuals with Factor IX deficiency.

Factor XI Deficiency

In Factor XI deficiency, the bleeding tendency varies among individuals and is often unrelated to the factor level. Menorrhagia is the frequent presenting syndrome in women. Spontenous bleeding is rare, but extensive hemorrhage can occur after trauma or surgery. Treatment with plasma to achieve a Factor XI level 30% of normal is adequate for normal hemostasis in most patients. DDAVP and antifibrinolytic agents may be considered for minor mucosal bleeding.[27]

Other Factor Deficiencies

Rarely, deficiencies of Factors V, X, VII, and XIII can cause bleeding diathesis. Because no factor concentrates are available for these factors, plasma products are used for replacement therapy. Patients with congenital Factor XII deficiency have no bleeding symptoms.

Alpha$_2$-Plasmin Inhibitor

Deficiency of alpha$_2$-plasmin inhibitor, the primary circulating plasmin inhibitor, is associated with a severe hemorrhagic disorder. Diagnosis requires a specific assay for this inhibitor. Therapy consists of replacement by plasma transfusion and/or oral antifibrinolytic agents such as epsilon aminocaproic acid.[28]

Acquired Bleeding Disorders

Patients with severe hemophilia A develop neutralizing IgG antibodies in 10% to 15% of cases after repeated Factor VIII infusions.[29]

In rare instances, spontaneous Factor VIII inhibitors occur as an autoimmune process in previously normal individuals. These autoantibodies are mainly seen in elderly patients with associated autoimmune or malignant disease or in younger women after childbirth. Patients usually present with severe bleeding. Therapy must be individualized, and it always requires consultation with a hematologist with expertise in the treatment of patients with inhibitors. Inhibitors to other coagulation factors occur very rarely.

Another acquired anticoagulant is the "lupus anticoagulant." It is a general term for a group of antibodies directed against a variety of phospholipid-binding proteins.[30] Prothrombin and beta-2 GPI are the most frequent antibody targets. These proteins interfere with the assembly of the coagulation factors on a phospholipid surface in vitro. Despite the prolongation of the aPTT and occasionally the PT in the test tube, these inhibitors are not associated with bleeding unless Factor II levels are also diminished, which may occur in rare cases. Paradoxically, these antibodies may be associated with thrombotic disorders, recurrent pregnancy loss, and thrombocytopenia.

The hallmark of an inhibitor is the incomplete correction of the prolonged clotting test using a 1:1 mixture of patient and normal plasma.

Heparin is one of the most frequently prescribed medications to treat or prevent venous thromboembolism (VTE). Heparin markedly enhances the ability of antithrombin to neutralize serine proteases. Even small amounts of heparin (eg, the flush volume in a subclavian catheter) can prolong the TT and the aPTT, leading to confusion in diagnosis. Heparin reversal is accomplished with protamine sulfate. Plasma is not effective in reversing heparin.

At the initiation of heparin therapy, the patient's platelet count should be closely monitored for the early detection of heparin-induced thrombocytopenia (HIT). In HIT, the platelet count falls to less than 50% of the pretreatment level or below 100,000/μL. This decrease occurs 5 to 15 days after initiation of therapy. Despite the low platelet count, thrombosis is the most feared complication. Heparin should be discontinued and alternative direct thrombin inhibitors (eg, hirudin, danaparin, argatroban) considered for anticoagulation.[31]

Vitamin K Deficiency and Antagonism: Vitamin K is a fat-soluble vitamin necessary for the synthesis in the liver of Factors II, VII, IX, and X; protein C; and protein S. Deficiency states can occur in patients in the intensive care unit, those who have chronic disease and are receiving antibiotics, and those with general fat malabsorption states, such as celiac disease, pancreatic insufficiency, or obstructive jaundice. The dose and route of administration depend on the clinical situation. Subcutaneous vitamin K corrects the deficiency in 6 to 12 hours. After oral administration of vitamin K, satisfactory reversal of anticoagulation can be achieved within 24 hours.[32] Intravenous infusion of vitamin K has been rarely associated with anaphylaxis, but a slow infusion rate reduces the risk. Urgent correction of deficiencies of the vitamin-K-dependent factors can be accomplished by plasma transfusions.

Oral anticoagulants, such as warfarin, work by interfering with vitamin-K-dependent synthesis of Factors II, VII, IX, and X. They also reduce the levels of the vitamin-K-dependent inhibitors, protein C and S. In rare cases, warfarin skin necrosis can develop about 4 days after initiation of therapy. Many, but not all patients, have concomitant protein C or protein S deficiency. Warfarin overdose is treated by withdrawal of the drug, administration of vitamin K, and, if bleeding is severe, by plasma transfusion. For emergent reversal of warfarin, activated vitamin K-dependent-factor concentrates (also called Prothrombin Complex Concentrates) can be used.

Liver Disease: Patients with liver disease have multiple coagulation derangements, including coagulation factor deficiencies, impaired vitamin K utilization, and activated fibrinolysis. Thrombocytopenia may add to the bleeding diathesis and is usually due to multiple factors including hypersplenism, increased platelet consumption, and diminished platelet production. Treatment with plasma is indicated in liver disease patients with a coagulopathy when bleeding is present, or when further dilution of coagulation factors is expected, from blood loss and replacement with red cells and plasma-free solutions. Prior to closed liver biopsy, paracentesis, and thoracentesis, patients with liver disease and a PT up to 1.5 times midrange of normal value did not have increased bleeding compared with those with a normal PT.[14,33] Patients with liver disease and mild coagulopathy are sensitive to dilutional coagulopathy. Plasma transfusion may be indicated in a bleeding patient to prevent or treat such dilution. The PT or an institutionally validated INR is suggested as a guideline for determining the hemostatic risk associated with factor deficiencies and need for plasma transfusion. It is important to note that correction of coagulation tests following plasma transfusion may not be complete due to the presence of fibrin fragments, dysfibrinogenemias, and rapid movement of factors into the extravascular space.

Disseminated Intravascular Coagulation: Uncontrolled activation of coagulation and secondary fibrinolysis causes disseminated intravascular coagulation (DIC). Thrombin is generated by pathologic release of tissue factor into the blood, or by widespread endothelial damage. Common clinical conditions predisposing to DIC include sepsis, trauma, obstetric complication, intravascular hemolysis, and malignancy. The chief clinical manifestation is bleeding in the acute form of DIC due to consumption of platelets and coagulation factors, mainly fibrinogen. In the chronic form of DIC, symptoms depend on the compensation capacity of the liver and marrow. The patient can present with singular or multiple thrombotic events or with low-grade bleeding. Routinely employed laboratory tests are neither sensitive nor specific for diagnosis of DIC. Serial measurement of PT, aPTT, platelet count, and fibrinogen level help to establish the diagnosis and guide therapy. Thrombocytopenia is present in 98% of cases. As the result of rapid fibrinolysis, fibrin degradation products and D-dimer levels increase. Vigorous treatment of the underlying disease and aggressive supportive measures are the cornerstones of therapy. Correction of bleeding may require transfusion of Platelets, Plasma, and/or Cryoprecipitated AHF. If thrombosis and tissue ischemia are prominent, heparin may be used to inhibit thrombin generation. Clinical trials demonstrate shortened duration of DIC with high-dose antithrombin therapy without clearly improved survival.[34] Recently, activated protein C concentrate was approved for the treatment of DIC secondary to sepsis. A hematologist should be consulted, especially if the use of these agents is contemplated.

Congenital Thrombophilia

Thrombophilia is a term used by clinicians to describe patients who develop venous or arterial thromboembolism spontaneously, at an early age, or at an unusual site or who have recurrent thrombotic events. It is multicausal and the majority of patients have several acquired and genetic risk factors.[35] The most common manifestation is deep vein thrombosis of the leg or pulmonary embolism. Testing for thrombophilia is best delayed for 1 month after anticoagulation has been completed. Molecular tests are not altered by anticoagulants.

Factor V Leiden Mutation

The most common inherited thrombophilic disorder is a mutation of Factor V. This mutation makes Factor V resistant to the inhibitory effect of activated protein C.[15] Between 1% and 8.5% of Caucasians are heterozygotes and the risk of venous thromboembolism is increased sevenfold. The relative risk in the homozygote is increased 80 times. The functional assay for detecting Factor V Leiden is activated protein C resistance test. Polymerase chain reaction is the most specific method to detect the nucleotide substitution (G1691A) responsible for this point mutation.

Prothrombin G20210A Mutation

This mutation in the 3'-untranslated region of the prothrombin gene is associated with elevated plasma prothrombin levels.[36] It is the second most frequent congenital risk factor for thrombosis. The gene is present in approximately 2% of Caucasians and in 6% of unselected patients with first thrombosis. It confers a nearly threefold risk for venous thromboembolism. There is no functional test for screening for this mutation, a method based on the polymerase chain reaction is used to detect carriers.

Patients who are double heterozygous for Factor V Leiden and prothrombin gene mutations have an over 40-fold increased risk of thrombosis. The co-inheritance of these two mutations is also associated with a higher risk of recurrence of thrombosis.[37]

Antithrombin Deficiency

Antithrombin potentiates the in-vivo effect of heparin. The prevalence of antithrombin deficiency in the general population is 0.02%. One percent of unselected patients with thrombosis have antithrombin deficiency. Family studies suggest that antithrombin

102

deficiency confers a higher risk for thrombosis than does a deficiency of protein C or protein S.[38]

Human-plasma-derived, virus-inactivated antithrombin concentrate (Thrombate III) is available. It is approved for patients with hereditary antithrombin deficiency in connection with surgery or pregnancy.

Protein C and Protein S Deficiencies

Heterozygous deficiencies of these two vitamin-K-dependent anticoagulant proteins are associated with recurrent thromboembolic disease. Homozygotes present with purpura fulminans as infants.[39] Diagnosis is established by specific assays. Protein C and S levels are diminished by oral anticoagulant therapy, which may obscure the diagnosis. Administration of warfarin therapy without prior heparinization may result in a sudden decrease of protein C and S in some patients with resultant warfarin skin necrosis. The prevalence of protein C deficiency is 0.2% to 0.3% in the general population; in unselected patients with venous thromboembolism it is around 3%. The prevalence of protein S deficiency is unknown. It is found in approximately 2% of patients with venous thromboembolism. Therapy for congenitally deficient patients is provided by plasma infusions.

Elevated Factor VIII

Sustained Factor VIII levels above 150 IU/dL are associated with a fivefold increased risk of venous thromboembolism compared to that seen when levels are less than 100 IU/dL. Factor VIII levels above 150 IU/dL have been found in 11% of the general population and 25% of patients with VTE.[40] Because it has a high prevalence and relative risk, the presence of elevated Factor VIII may be responsible for more thrombotic events than was previously appreciated.

Disorders of Fibrinolysis

Primary disorders of fibrinolysis are rare and hard to differentiate from DIC. Most fibrinolytic states are secondary to strong procoagulant stimuli. Antifibrinolytic therapy (eg, EACA or aprotinin) has been reported to be successful in the treatment of bleeding states associated with an activated fibrinolytic mechanism, such as cardiopulmonary bypass procedures and liver transplantation. EACA and tranexamic acid are useful as adjunct therapy with factor replacement in bleeding disorders particularly during and after dental procedures. Use of EACA should never be undertaken without hematologic consultation, because blockade of the fibrinolytic system can be associated with pathologic thrombosis.

The therapeutic administration of the plasminogen activators streptokinase and urokinase, or of recombinant tissue-type plasminogen activator has grown increasingly important in the treatment of thrombotic disease. These agents may be used locally (ie, infused via angiographic control directly into the thrombosed area) or systemically (via peripheral vein). Successful results have been reported in deep-vein thrombosis, intra-abdominal thrombosis, thrombosis at the site of indwelling catheters, pulmonary embolism, and in peripheral and coronary arterial occlusions. Contraindications to therapy include recent cranial trauma or known intracranial lesions, and recent major surgery. Laboratory monitoring is not precise, and treatment regimens are standardized for each agent. The lytic state can be monitored by periodic assay of fibrinogen concentration or the thrombin time. Uncontrolled bleeding due to these agents should be treated by discontinuation of the drug, repletion of fibrinogen with cryoprecipitate, and, in extreme cases, with inhibitors of fibrinolysis.

References

1. NIH consensus development conference. Platelet transfusion therapy. JAMA 1987;257:1777-80.

2. Fresh-Frozen Plasma, Cryoprecipitate and Platelets Administration Practice Guidelines Development Task Force of the College of American Pathologists. Practice parameter for the use of fresh frozen plasma, cryoprecipitate, and platelets. JAMA 1994;271:777-81.

3. Gmur J, Burger J, Schanz U, et al. Safety of stringent prophylactic platelet transfusion policy for patients with acute leukaemia. Lancet 1991;338:1223-6.

4. Rebulla P, Finazzi G, Marangoni F, et al. A multicenter randomized study of the threshold for prophylactic platelet transfusions in adults with acute myeloid leukemia. Gruppo Italiano Malattie Ematolotgiche Maligne. N Engl J Med 1997:337:1870-5.

5. Norol F, Kuentz M, Cordonnier C, et al. Influence of clinical status on the efficiency of stored platelet transfusion. Br J Haematol 1994;86:125-9.

6. Alcorta I, Pereira A, Ordinas A. Clinical and laboratory factors associated with platelet transfusion refractoriness: A case-control study. Br J Haematol 1996;93:220-4.

7. Gewirtz AS, Miller ML, Keys TF. The clinical usefulness of the preoperative bleeding time. Arch Pathol Lab Med 1996;120(4):353-6.

8. Peterson P, Hayes TE, Arkin CF, et al. The preoperative bleeding time test lacks clinical benefit: College of American Pathologists' and American Society of Clinical Pathologists' position article. Arch Surg 1998;133(2):134-9.

9. Mammen EF, Comp PC, et al. PFA-100 system: A new method for assessment of platelet dysfunction. Semin Thromb Hemost 1998;24:195-202.

10. Ortel TL, James AH, Thames EH, et al. Assessment of primary Hemostasis by PFA-100 analysis in a tertiary care center. Thromb Haemost 2000;84:93-7.

11. Chew DP, Moliterno DJ. A critical appraisal of platelet glycoprotein IIb/IIIa inhibition. J Am Coll Cardiol 2000; 36:2028-35.

12. Jubelirer SJ, Koenig BA, Bates MC. Acute profound thrombocytopenia following c7E3 Fab (abciximab) therapy: Case reports, review of the literature and implications for therapy. Am J Hematol 1999;61:205-8.

13. Dahlback B. Blood coagulation. Lancet 2000;355: 1627-32.

14. McVay PA, Toy PTCY. Lack of increased bleeding after liver biopsy in patients with mild hemostatis abnormalities. Am J Clin Pathol 1990;94:747-53.

15. Dahlback B. Resistance to activated protein C caused by the factor V R506Q mutation is a common risk factor for venous thrombosis. Thromb Haemost 1997;78(1):P483-8.

16. van Tilburg NH, Rosendaal FR, Bertina RM. Thrombin activable fibrinolysis inhibitor and the risk for deep vein thrombosis. Blood 2000;95:2855-9.

17. Mallett SV, Cox DJA. Thrombelastography. Br J Anaesth 1992;69(3);307-13.

18. Carr JM, Kruskall MS, Kaye JA, Robinson SH. Efficacy of platelet transfusions in immune thrombocytopenia. Am J Med 1986;80:1051-4.

19. Gordon LI, Kwaan HC, Rossi EC. Deleterious effects of platelet transfusions and recovery thrombocytosis in patients with thrombotic microangiopathy. Semin Hematol 1987;24:194-201.

20. The Trial to Reduce Alloimmunization to Platelets Study Group. Leukocyte reduction and ultraviolet B irradiation of platelets to prevent alloimmunization and refractoriness to platelet transfusions. N Engl J Med 1997;337:1861-9.

21. Weigert AL, SchaferAI. Uremic bleeding: Pathogenesis and therapy. Am J Med Sci 1998, 316(2):94-104.

22. Sadler JE, Gralnick HR. Commentary. A new classification for von Willebrand disease. Blood 1994;84:676-9.

23. Mannucci PM. How I treat patients with von Willebrand disease. Blood 2001;97:1915-16.

24. Hambleton J. Advances in the treatment of von Willebrand disease. Semin Hematol 2001:38(suppl 9);7-10.

25. Mannucci PM, Edward GD, Tuddenham MD. The hemophilias—from royal genes to gene therapy. N Eng J Med 2001;344:1773-9.

26. Mikaelsson M, Oswaldsson U, Sandberg H. Influence of phospholipids on the assessment of factor VIII activity. Haemophilia 1998;4:646-50.

27. Bolton-Maggs PH. Bleeding problems in factor XI deficient women. Haemophilia 1999;5:155-9.

28. Favier R, Aoki N, De Moerloose P. Congenital alpha-2-plasmin inhibitor deficiencies: A review. Br J Haematol 2001;114:4-10.

29. Engelfriet CP, Reesink HW. The optimal treatment for haemophiliacs who have developed factor VIII or -IX antibodies. Vox Sang 2000;78:256-61.

30. Arnout J. Antiphospholipid syndrome: Diagnostic aspect of lupus anticoagulants. Thromb Haemost 2001;86:83-91.

31. Fabris F, Ahmad S, Cella G, et al. Pathophysiology of heparin-induced thrombocytopenia. Clinical and diagnostic implications—a review. Arch Pathol Lab Med 2000;124:1657-66.

32. Watson HG, Baglin T, Laidlaw SL, et al. A comparison of the efficacy and rate of response to oral and intravenous vitamin K reversal of over-anticoagulation with warfarin. Br J Haematol 2001;115:145-9.

33. McVay PA, Toy PTCY. Lack of increased bleeding after paracentesis and thoracentesis in patients with mild coagulation abnormalities. Transfusion 1991;31:164-71.

34. Riewald M, Riess H. Treatment options for clinically recognized DIC. Semin Throm Hemost 1998;24:53-9.

35. Mannucci PM The molecular basis of inherited thrombophilia. Vox Sang 2000;78(2 suppl):39-45.

36. Poort SR, Rosendaal FR, Reitsma PH, Bertina RM. A common genetic variation in the 3-untranslated region of the prothrombin gene is associated with elevated prothrombin levels and an increase in venous thrombosis. Blood 1996;88:3698-703.

37. Margaglione M, D'Andrea G, Colaizzo D, et al. Coexistence of factor V Leiden and Factor II A20210 mutations and recurrent thromboembolism. Thromb Haemost 1999;82:1583-7.

38. Rosendaal FR. Risk factors for venous thrombotic disease. Thromb Haemostasis 1999;82:616-9.

39. Clonse LH, Comp PC. The regulation of hemostasis: The protein C system. N Engl J Med 1986;314:1298-304.

40. Koster T, Blann AD, Briet E, Vandenbrouke JP, Rosendaal FR. Role of clotting factor VIII in effect of von Willebrand factor on occurrence of deep-vein thrombosis. Lancet 1995;345:152-5.

ADVERSE EFFECTS OF BLOOD TRANSFUSION

Acute Transfusion Reactions

Blood transfusions can cause untoward reactions in as many as 10% of recipients. Because of this risk, transfusion should be administered only when the benefits clearly outweigh the risks. Patients should be advised of the risks, benefits, alternatives to, and consequences of refusal of transfusion. Documentation of informed consent is required.

Acute transfusion reactions occur during or within 24 hours after a transfusion. Most life-threatening transfusion reactions occur early in the course of transfusion; therefore, all patients should be carefully monitored throughout transfusion and any adverse signs and symptoms should be promptly investigated. It is important to recognize that acute reactions may occur after a transfusion is completed. If a reaction occurs during the course of a multiple unit transfusion, the unit currently being transfused may not necessarily be the cause of the reaction.

Acute Hemolytic Reactions

Hemolytic transfusion reactions (HTRs) are caused by the immune-mediated lysis of transfused red cells. Such reactions can be acute or delayed, and result in intravascular or extravascular hemolysis. An acute hemolytic transfusion reaction (AHTR) occurs when incompatible red cells are transfused to a recipient who already has a clinically significant preformed antibody to an antigen present on the transfused cells, such as transfusion of group A red cells into a group O or a group B recipient. Patient misidentification, occurring either when the blood specimen for compatibility testing is drawn or when a transfusion is administered, is the most common cause of ABO-incompatible transfusion, resulting is acute hemolysis. AHTRs occur typically within minutes of the start of the infusion. If the recipient's antibody fixes complement, as most often occurs with ABO-incompatible blood transfusions, an acute intravascular hemolytic transfusion reaction (AIHTR) results.[1] The anti-A and anti-B responsible are either IgM or complement-fixing IgG, both of which activate complement resulting in the binding of the C5-9 component of complement (the membrane attack complex). Fixation of C5-9 results in the appearance of a pore in the red cell membrane. Water enters the cell through this channel and osmotic intravascular lysis results. This produces hemoglobinemia and, as free hemoglobin is cleared by the kidney, hemoglobinuria. These two signs are critical for the diagnosis of an AIHTR. Characteristic laboratory findings in AHTR may also include decreased hematocrit, decreased haptoglobin, increased lactate dehydrogenase (LDH), and the presence of plasma hemoglobin. Serum bilirubin typically increases 6 to 12 hours later.

The severe clinical symptoms of shock, hypotension, and bronchospasm seen in an AIHTR are due to the generated complement fragments, anaphylatoxins C3a and C5a, and to other mediators of inflammation.[2,3] In addition, renal ischemia occurs, which may result in tubular necrosis and the development of acute renal failure. Binding of nitric oxide by free hemoglobin exacerbates renal ischemia. Nitric oxide, known as endothelium-derived relaxing factor (EDRF), is a potent vasodilator. EDRF activity is balanced by endothelin, a potent vasoconstrictor. Binding of nitric oxide thus promotes renal vasoconstriction, tubular necrosis, and renal failure.[3] The coagulation cascade may be activated as well, initiating disseminated intravascular coagulation (DIC). Clinical symptoms are in large part attributable to activation of the cytokine network, including the proinflammatory cytokines interleukin-1 (IL-1), IL-6, IL-8, and tumor necrosis factor-alpha (TNF-α), which produce fever, hypotension, and activation of white cells and the clotting cascade.[4,5]

The severity of AIHTR depends on the rate and amount of blood transfused. Generally, the more incompatible blood given and the faster the infusion rate, the more severe the reaction. Treatment of an AIHTR, a medical emergency, is described in Table 4. If an AIHTR is suspected, infusion of the unit should be stopped immediately and additional units of red cells should not be administered until the cause has been identified and corrected. When transfusion is urgent, communication with the blood bank is critical. The occurrence of acute intravascular hemolysis in the absence of red cell incompatibility should prompt the search for a nonimmunologic etiology for hemolysis (see below).

While most AHTRs are intravascular, if the antibody does not fix complement, or fixes only to C3, the resulting reaction will be an acute extravascular HTR (Table 5). Acute extravascular HTRs (AEHTRs) are not associated with the serious clinical symptom complex seen in Table 5, because there is much less generation of the biologic response modifiers such as C3a, C5a and the cytokines IL-1, IL-6, and other proinflammatory cytokines.[6] AEHTRs typically present with fever, a new positive direct antiglobulin test (DAT) result due to antibody binding to the *transfused* incompatible red cells, and a falling hematocrit without any overt signs of bleeding. Hemoglobinemia and hemoglobinuria are rarely seen in an AEHTR due to the lack of fixation of the C5-9 complement complex to the red cell membrane. The passive infusion of incompatible isohemagglutinins, which may occur with transfusion of the plasma contained in ABO-incompatible platelets, and rarely intravenous immune globulin (IVIG), can cause severe hemolytic reactions.[7-9]

Sickle Cell Hemolytic Transfusion Reaction Syndrome

Patients with sickle cell disease are at high risk for HTRs because of frequent transfusion and phenotype differences from the donor population. HTRs in sickle cell disease can precipitate a hemolytic crisis and result in a greater degree of anemia than before transfusion, resulting from bystander hemolysis of autologous red cells. This phenomenon has been termed the sickle cell hemolytic transfusion reaction syndrome.[10] In this syndrome, the corrected

Table 4. Workup of an Acute Transfusion Reaction

If an acute transfusion reaction occurs:
1. Stop blood component transfusion immediately
2. Verify the correct unit was given to the correct patient
3. Maintain IV access and ensure adequate urine output with an appropriate crystalloid or colloid solution
4. Maintain blood pressure and pulse
5. Maintain adequate ventilation
6. Notify attending physician and blood bank
7. Obtain blood/urine for transfusion reaction workup
8. Send report of reaction, samples, blood bag, and administration set to blood bank
9. Blood bank performs workup of suspected transfusion reaction as follows:
   A. A clerical check is performed to ensure correct blood component was transfused to the right patient
   B. The plasma is visually evaluated for hemoglobinemia
   C. A direct antiglobulin test is performed
   D. Other serologic testing is repeated as needed (ABO, Rh, crossmatch)

If intravascular hemolytic reaction is confirmed:
1. Monitor renal status (BUN, creatinine)
2. Initiate a diuresis. Avoid fluid overload if renal failure is present.
3. Analyze urine for hemoglobinuria
4. Monitor coagulation status (PT, aPTT, fibrinogen, platelet count)
5. Monitor for signs of hemolysis (LDH, bilirubin, haptoglobin, plasma hemoglobin)
6. Monitor hemoglobin and hematocrit
7. Repeat compatibility testing (crossmatch)
8. **Consult with blood bank physician before further transfusion.**

If bacterial contamination is suspected:
1. Obtain blood culture of patient
2. Return unit or empty blood bag to blood bank for culture and Gram's stain
3. Maintain circulation and urine output
4. Initiate broad spectrum antibiotic treatment as appropriate; revise antibiotic regimen based on microbiological results
5. Monitor for signs of DIC, renal failure, respiratory failure.

Adapted from Snyder EL. Transfusion reactions. In: Hoffman R, Benz EF Jr, Shattil SJ, et al. Hematology: Basic principles and practice, 2nd ed. New York: Churchill Livingstone, 1995;2045-53.

Table 5. Acute Transfusion Reactions

Type	Signs and Symptoms	Usual Cause	Treatment	Prevention
Intravascular hemolytic (immune)	Hemoglobinemia and hemoglobinuria, fever, chills, anxiety, shock, DIC, dyspnea, chest pain, flank pain, oliguria	ABO incompatibility (clerical error) or other complement-fixing red cell antibody	Stop transfusion; hydrate, support blood pressure and respiration; induce diuresis; treat shock and DIC, if present	Ensure proper sample and recipient identification
Extravascular hemolytic (immune)	Fever, malaise, indirect hyperbilirubinemia, increased LDH, urine urobilinogen, falling hematocrit	IgG non-complement-fixing antibody	Monitor hematocrit, renal and hepatic function, coagulation profile; no acute treatment generally required	Review historical records; ensure proper sample and recipient identification; give antigen-negative units as appropriate; possible high-dose IVIG

(Continued)

Table 5. Acute Transfusion Reactions (Continued)

Type	Signs and Symptoms	Usual Cause	Treatment	Prevention
Febrile	Fever, chills	Antibodies to leukocytes or plasma proteins; hemolysis; passive cytokine infusion; bacterial contamination; commonly due to patient's underlying condition	Stop transfusion; give antipyretics, eg, acetaminophen; for rigors in adults use meperidine 25 to 50 mg IV or IM	Pretransfusion antipyretic; leukocyte-reduced blood components
Allergic (mild to severe)	Urticaria (hives), dyspnea, wheezing, throat tightening, rarely hypotension or anaphylaxis	Antibodies to plasma proteins; rarely antibodies to IgA	Stop transfusion; give antihistamine (PO or IM); if severe, epinephrine and/or steroids	Pretransfusion antihistamine; washed RBC, if recurrent or severe; check pretransfusion IgA levels in patients with a history of anaphylaxis to transfusion
Hypotension	Hypotension, tachycardia	Bradykinin generation, may be exacerbated by ACE inhibitor	Stop transfusion; fluids; Trendelenberg position	Discontinue ACE inhibitor; avoid bedside leukocyte reduction filters

Hypervolemia	Dyspnea, hypertension, pulmonary edema, cardiac arrhythmias	Too rapid and/or excessive blood transfusion	Induce diuresis; phlebotomy; support cardiorespiratory system as needed	Avoid rapid or excessive transfusion
Transfusion-related acute lung injury (TRALI)	Dyspnea, fever, hypoxia pulmonary edema, hypotension, normal pulmonary capillary wedge pressure	Donor HLA or leukocyte antibody transfused with plasma in component; less commonly recipient antibody to donor white cells; neutrophil-priming lipid mediator	Support blood pressure and respiration (may require intubation)	Leukocyte-reduced RBCs and platelets; notify transfusion service and blood center to test donors(s) quarantine remaining components from donor(s)
Bacterial contamination	Rigors, chills, fever, shock	Contaminated blood component	Stop transfusion; support blood pressure; culture patient and blood unit; give antibiotics; notify blood transfusion service	Care in donor selection, blood collection and storage; careful attention to arm-preparation for phlebotomy

DIC = disseminated intravascular coagulation; IV = intravenous; IM = intramuscular; PO = by mouth; RBC = red blood cells; ACE = angiotensin converting enzyme reticulocyte count and absolute number of hemoglobin-S-containing red cells increase during the reaction.[10,11] Pain crisis in a sickle cell patient following transfusion should suggest the occurrence of sickle cell hemolytic transfusion reaction syndrome. Further transfusion in this setting may exacerbate the anemia, and even prove fatal. Serologic studies may not provide a clear explanation for HTR in these patients. Patients on a hypertransfusion protocol may have suppressed erythropoiesis that obscures the diagnosis. In addition, the presence of multiple alloantibodies may make the serologic diagnosis difficult.

Drug-Induced Hemolysis

Many drugs can induce production of antibodies against red cells and cause hemolysis. While drug-induced hemolysis is not a transfusion reaction, it can be readily confused with HTR in the transfused patient. Most drugs that cause hemolysis induce a neo-antigen on the red cell membrane, either through a hapten mechanism or by modification of membrane proteins. Some drugs induce the formation of immune complexes in plasma that deposit on the red cell surface and result in accelerated clearance. Rarely, a drug may induce an autoantibody to red cells. In drug-induced hemolysis both autologous and transfused red cells will be eliminated. Typically, there is a positive DAT result and the serum will react with red cells in the presence, but not the absence, of the offending drug. Clinically, drug-induced hemolysis may be indistinguishable from AHTR. The hemolysis may be severe and even fatal. Treatment consists of discontinuing the drug, supportive care, and transfusion to maintain adequate oxygen-carrying capacity. Presently, the cephalosporin antibiotics, cefotetan, and ceftriaxone are the most common causes of drug-induced immune hemolysis.[12]

Nonimmune Hemolysis

Mechanical hemolysis of transfused blood can occur with artificial heart valves, with extracorporeal circulation, or transfusion through small-bore catheters under high pressure because of the shear stress imposed on erythrocytes. Administration of hypotonic saline solutions, 5% dextrose in water (D5W), distilled water, or certain medications in the same line as the blood infusion can result in osmotic lysis of transfused red cells. Heating above 42 C due to a malfunctioning blood warmer, or freezing due to exposure to ice or a refrigerator malfunction, may hemolyze blood prior to transfusion. Although hemoglobinuria may occur in nonimmune hemolysis, it is rarely associated with the symptom complex seen with AHTR. Transfusion of hemolyzed blood can cause hyperkalemia and transient renal impairment. However, the cause of hemoglobinemia and/or hemoglobinuria must be evaluated as soon as possible, because delay in the recognition of an immune AHTR could lead to serious clinical complications.

Febrile Nonhemolytic Transfusion Reactions

Fever is a common symptom of a transfusion reaction (Table 5), and may be the first sign of a febrile (fever-chill) reaction, bacterial contamination, or an AHTR. Fever results from the production of pyrogens (IL-1, IL-6, and TNF-α) that act on the thermoregulatory center in the hypothalamus through the intermediary of prostaglandin E2. Fever may be caused by the patient's underlying condition; thus fever, per se, is not a contraindication for administering a blood transfusion. A febrile nonhemolytic transfusion reaction (FNHTR) is defined as temperature rise of greater than 1 C (1.8 F), typically accompanied by chills or rigors occurring during or up to 2 hours after a transfusion, that is not attributable to another cause. The incidence of FNHTRs, while less than 1% in infrequently transfused recipients, has historically been reported in up to 10% of chronically transfused patients. Febrile reactions may be attributed to antibodies directed against transfused leukocytes or platelets. The resulting antigen-antibody reactions trigger phagocytes to release endogenous pyrogens, causing fever.[4,13] Alternatively, leukocytes in cellular blood components may produce pyrogens during storage.[14] The use of leukocyte-reduced blood components can mitigate, but not necessarily eliminate, these reactions.[15,16] Because pyrogenic cytokines may be produced by events unrelated to the transfusion, the diagnosis of FNHTR is one of exclusion. Transfusion of stored blood components containing preformed cytokines may explain why some patients experience FNHTRs despite the use of third-generation blood filters at issue or at the bedside. Pyrogenic cytokines contained in the plasma of stored Platelets have been shown to cause fever, independent of the cellular portion.[17] The removal of plasma from stored Platelets decreases, but does not eliminate, the incidence of febrile reactions. Prestorage leukocyte reduction can eliminate the accumulation of pryogens.[18] There is controversy regarding whether prestorage leukocyte reduction decreases the incidence of febrile reactions, though the preponderance of evidence suggests that it does.[19,20] Another postulated mechanism for FNHTR is that during storage platelets also release CD40 ligand (CD154), which can stimulate endothelial cells to produce prostaglandin E2 in a manner similar to pyrogenic cytokines.[21]

Most febrile reactions respond to antipyretics. In general, aspirin should not be used in thrombocytopenic patients. For such patients, acetaminophen, or nonsteroidal anti-inflammatory agents are preferred. Febrile reactions are rarely serious, although rigors can be a significant stress for a patient with compromised cardiorespiratory status. Rigors may be treated with meperidine, although it should be used with caution in patients with impaired respiratory drive. Antihistamines do not prevent febrile reactions and have no role in prophylaxis.

Allergic Reactions

Allergic reactions occur in about 1% of all transfusion recipients, but are more frequent in heavily transfused patients. They are likely caused by antigen-antibody reactions that result from the infusion of plasma proteins. The signs and symptoms may vary from localized cutaneous manifestations (urticaria, flushing, itching, and sometimes mild fever) to systemic symptoms of nausea, vomiting, diarrhea, and bronchospasm. Rarely, frank anaphylactic reactions occur. A patient who develops mild allergic reactions (eg, localized hives) will not progress to more severe anaphylactic reactions with additional infusion of blood; the severity of an allergic reaction is not usually dose-related. Most allergic reactions are mild, do not recur, and respond to oral or parenteral antihistamines. With mild, localized reactions, the transfusion may be continued after medication is given, provided the signs and symptoms subside. If only hives have developed, the risk associated with restarting the transfusion is less than the already small risk of transfusion-transmitted diseases associated with an additional donor exposure. It is stressed that this applies only to mild allergic transfusion reactions and not to reactions in patients presenting with fever, chills, dyspnea, wheezing, laryngeal edema, or anaphylaxis. Leukocyte reduction of components does not prevent allergic reactions. Anaphylactic reactions can be caused by antibodies to IgA, haptoglobin, or C4 (Chido/Rogers blood group antigens).[22-24] For severe allergic or anaphylactic reactions, the transfusion should be stopped immediately, and IV access should be secured while fluid resuscitation and treatment with epinephrine and/or steroids is started. Severe reactions may require treatment with vasopressors and intubation, as would treatment of any anaphylactic reaction. When further transfusion is indicated, washed cellular blood components should be considered.[25] Transfusion of components containing plasma to such patients presents a difficult problem that requires careful risk/benefit analysis. Pretransfusion treatment with high-dose corticosteroids and antihistamines should be considered, and immediate availability of epinephrine should be ensured. A typical dose schedule is to premedicate the patient 30 to 60 minutes prior to transfusion with 100 mg of hydrocortisone given intravenously and 25 to 50 mg of diphenhydramine given orally or parenterally. IgA-deficient individuals may require IgA-deficient plasma that can be obtained through rare donor registries.

Circulatory Overload

Hypervolemia (circulatory overload) develops when the patient is unable to compensate for expanded blood volume. Signs and symptoms of circulatory overload include headache, shortness of breath, pulmonary edema, congestive heart failure, and systolic hypertension (>50 mmHg rise). Symptoms usually subside if the transfusion is stopped, the patient is placed in a sitting position, and given oxygen and diuretics to remove fluid. If symptoms persist, a phlebotomy may be necessary. Rarely, hypertension with volume overload can lead to flash pulmonary edema. To avoid hypervolemia, blood components should not be infused at a rate faster than 2 to 4 mL/kg/hour. Slower rates are needed for patients at risk of fluid overload, such as patients with chronic anemia who have an expanded plasma volume, or patients with compromised cardiac and/or pulmonary function. In these situations, aliquots from a single unit of blood can be transfused slowly over time, not to exceed 4 hours.

Transfusion-Related Acute Lung Injury

Transfusion-related acute lung injury (TRALI) manifests as noncardiogenic pulmonary edema during or shortly after transfusion. It is differentiated from circulatory overload by the lack of heart failure.[26] The passive transfer of high titer anti-HLA or white cell antibody (leukoagglutinins) directed against recipient leukocytes has been associated with a spectrum of acute lung injuries that manifest as acute pulmonary edema. This reaction results from activation of recipient neutrophils in the lungs with the production of vasoactive mediators ultimately causing capillary leakage. Infusion of HLA or granulocyte-specific antibody in plasma-containing components, reacting with a recipient antigen, is the most common cause of this reaction. The donor of the implicated unit is often a multiparous woman.[27] Less commonly, recipient antibodies directed against donor leukocytes are implicated as a cause of TRALI. Alternatively, a lipid mediator produced by donor leukocytes during storage may prime recipient neutrophils so that a second stimulus, such as inflammation, infection or tissue injury, results in the release of vasoactive medicators (the two-hit hypothesis).[28] In its full form, TRALI presents as marked respiratory distress, hypoxia, hypotension, fever, and bilateral pulmonary edema occurring during or within 4 hours of a transfusion.[26] However, milder forms of TRALI occur that may be difficult to recognize as such. These reactions typically resolve within 48 to 72 hours, although the mortality rate is approximately 10%. Leuko-cyte-reduced components are indicated for subsequent transfusions, because the reaction may be due to recipient HLA antibodies. The treatment of TRALI reactions is supportive. The patient may require supplemental oxygen, endotracheal intubation, and respiratory support until the intra-alveolar fluid can be resorbed. Diuresis is not indicated. Steroids may shorten the course of TRALI, but their role in therapy is not clear. Fluid support may be necessary for resuscitation in the event of hypotension and marked movement of fluid from plasma to the extravascular space. Suspected TRALI reactions should be reported to the blood supplier to ascertain information about the donor(s) of the transfused blood components and to prompt the quarantine or recall of additional components from the donor(s). A test for HLA and leukocyte antibodies in donor plasma and, if positive, HLA antigen typing of the recipient may help establish the diagnosis.

Hypotensive Reactions to Transfusion

Hypotensive reactions following some platelet and red cell transfusions have been reported and appear to involve generation of bradykinin from activation of the kinin pathway caused by contact of plasma with artificial surfaces. Bradykinin is a potent vasodilator that causes hypotension, abdominal pain, and facial flushing.[29-31] Some of these reactions have occurred in patients receiving blood through a negatively charged bedside leukocyte reduction filter, while medicated with angiotensin-converting enzyme (ACE) inhibitor drugs. ACE is identical to kininase II, the principal enzyme that degrades bradykinin. Inhibition of kininase II prolongs the half-life of bradykinin in these patients and can worsen the clinical symptomatology. Because bradykinin has a half-life of 15 to 30 seconds, prestorage leukocyte reduction rather than bedside leukocyte reduction should eliminate reactions caused by contact with the filter biomaterials. Transfusion-associated hypotension typically resolves within minutes of stopping the transfusion. These reactions must be differentiated from vasovagal reactions, AHTR, bacterial contamination, and anaphylaxis.

Bacterial Contamination

Bacterial contamination of stored blood poses a rare but serious risk to the transfusion recipient. Bacteria can enter a blood bag due to improper preparation of the skin at the venipuncture site at the time of phlebotomy, during component preparation or handling, or because of occult bacteremia in the donor. The overall rate of bacterial contamination of blood collections determined by prospective culture has been reported to be 0.3%, although the incidence of serious reactions is less.[32] Skin flora (Staphylococcus, Propionibacteria) are the most common isolates from prospectively cultured units, but other species are more often implicated in clinical reactions. Gram-negative rods (*Acinetobacter, Klebsiella, Escherichia*) are more common than gram-positive cocci (*Staphylococcus, Strepto-coccus*) in reactions to contaminated RBC and Platelets.[33] Bacteria capable of growing at low temperature in a high iron environment, *Yersinia* or *Pseudomonas,* may proliferate in RBC units. Contaminated units of RBCs may appear normal to visual inspection or may appear dark or contain clots. During or after the transfusion, the patient may develop rigors, high fever, dyspnea, hypotension, and shock. Hemoglobinemia and hemoglobinuria are usually absent. It is essential that any transfusion in progress be stopped when a contaminated unit is suspected. Aggressive resuscitative therapy and broad-spectrum antibiotics should be started immediately when a septic transfusion reaction is considered. Suspected septic transfusion reactions should be immediately reported to the transfusion service, because additional components from the same donation could be infected and must be recalled. These components could produce similar or even more severe reactions in other recipients. The suspected unit should be evaluated with Gram's stain and cultured. Septic reactions may not manifest until several hours after the transfusion of a unit of contaminated blood. Although rare, septic transfusion reactions can be fatal.

Thermal Effects

The rapid transfusion of blood directly from refrigerator storage can result in hypothermia with resultant cardiac arrythmia or arrest. Conversely, over-warming blood can also produce hemolysis. Blood should only be warmed using a monitored blood warming system. Warming blood with unmonitored out-of-the-faucet hot tap water, or in an unmonitored microwave device is unacceptable.

Metabolic Complications

Blood is anticoagulated with citrate, which chelates calcium ions. If citrated blood is infused rapidly and the ionized calcium level falls transiently, the patient may complain of tingling around the mouth (circumoral paresthesia) and in the fingers.[34] These symptoms subside quickly if the transfusion is slowed because citrate is rapidly metabolized by patients with normal liver function. Under no circumstances should calcium be added to a unit of blood, as it could reverse the anticoagulant effect of the citrate, producing large blood clots.

During storage of RBCs there is reversible leakage of potassium into the supernatant. Although the potassium concentration may be high, the total amount of potassium in a unit of RBCs is usually inconsequential. Hyperkalemia due to the massive infusion of stored blood is rare. Hyperkalemia may be a concern in neonates, especially in the context of exchange transfusion, and sometimes in liver transplantation, pediatric cardiac surgery, and in some patients with renal failure. Washing of RBCs, removal of the supernatant, or use of blood less than 7 days old can be helpful in such cases. With large-volume transfusion, the production of bicarbonate from the infused citrate more often produces an alkalosis, resulting in hypokalemia, which may actually require potassium administration.[35]

Delayed Transfusion Reactions

Delayed Hemolytic Reactions

Delayed hemolytic transfusion reactions (DHTRs) occur when transfused red cells induce an antibody response in a recipient days or weeks after the transfusion episode. The difference in the time of antibody production relates to whether it is an anamnestic response (days) or a primary response (weeks) to transfusion. It has been estimated that with each unit of blood transfused, there is a 1% to 1.6% risk of sensitizing a recipient to a red cell antigen other than the D antigen.[36] Most DHTRs are extravascular, and they are often associated with antibodies to Rh and Kell system antigens. Because the antibodies involved in a delayed extravascular hemolytic transfusion reactions rarely fix complement, the clinical signs and symptoms are usually much less severe than those associated with AHTRs. IgG-mediated phagocytosis results in inflammatory cytokine production, but at a lower level than in AHTR.[6] Due to the low level of inflammatory response and lack of complement activation, patients with DEHTRs often manifest only slight fever, malaise, weakness, and symptoms referable to anemia. A positive DAT result will be caused by the coating of the transfused donor red cells with recipient antibody. Destruction of the transfused red cells may cause anemia and indirect hyperbilirubinemia. Other laboratory findings may include an elevated reticulocyte count, increased LDH, and decreased haptoglobin. Hemoglobinemia is unusual. In rare situations were transfusion is necessary, but compatible blood is not obtainable, high-dose IVIG (400 mg/kg) given before transfusion may prevent DEHTR.[37]

Delayed intravascular hemolytic transfusion reactions also occur, often associated with antibodies to the Duffy (Fy^a, Fy^b) or Kidd (Jk^a or Jk^b) blood group antigen systems. While the C5-9 component of complement may be fixed to the red cell membrane and hemolysis with hemoglobinemia and hemoglobinuria may occur, the rate of generation of C3a, C5a, proinflammatory cytokines, and other biologic response modifiers is lower than in an *acute* IHTR and thus, the clinical symptoms in a *delayed* IHTR are rarely life-threatening. If a patient shows signs of a severe transfusion reaction, however, treatment should follow that described for an AIHTR. Delayed hemolytic reactions are also observed in ABO- and Rh-mismatched hematopoietic cell and solid organ transplants.

Posttransfusion Purpura

Posttransfusion purpura (PTP) is characterized by the onset of profound thrombocytopenia 1 to 3 weeks after transfusion. All types of blood components have been implicated in PTP. In these reactions, there is an alloantibody response to a platelet antigen. Most cases have been associated with antibodies to the HPA-1a antigen on the glycoprotein IIb/IIIa complex, but other platelet antigens have also been implicated as well. The diagnosis is established by the finding of a platelet-specific antibody in an antigen-negative patient. The thrombocytopenia of PTP typically persists for 2 to 3 weeks and resolves spontaneously without treatment. The most likely pathophysiologic explanation for PTP is that early in the course of an alloimmune response, the patient produces low-affinity antibodies that cross-react with autologous platelets. As the immune response naturally matures, low-affinity cross-reacting clones are eliminated and a pure alloantibody remains. The treatment of PTP is dependent on the clinical picture. Stable patients with low risk of hemorrhage may be followed closely until the platelet count returns to normal. Patients with significant bleeding or risk of hemorrhage should receive treatment to shorten the course of thrombocytopenia. High-dose Immune Globulin (400 to 500 mg/kg) has been reported to increase the platelet count abruptly.[38] Alternatively, plasmapheresis may be used to remove the causative antibody.[39] Platelet transfusion is indicated for severe bleeding, but prophylactic platelet transfusion is futile. There is no utility in transfusing antigen-negative platelets, even when a specificity is identified, because that patient is destroying perfectly matched platelets, his own. Steroids have not been shown to shorten the course of PTP.

Graft-vs-Host Disease

Graft-vs-host disease (GVHD), a well-recognized complication of allogeneic hematopoietic cell transplantation, can also occur after the transfusion of immunologically competent donor lymphocytes, usually to an immunoincompetent recipient.[40,41] Transfusion-associated GVHD (TA-GVHD) also has been observed after transfusion of cellular components from HLA-homozygous donors to immunocompetent recipients who are heterozygous for the HLA haplotype.[42] While the latter occurs more frequently after transfusion of blood from first- or second-degree relatives, it has been reported to occur with transfusion of blood from unrelated HLA-homozygous donors.[43] GVHD is initiated by alloreactive donor T cells recognizing host histocompatibility antigens.[44] Donor lymphocytes engraft in the recipient, proliferate, and attack host tissue. TA-GVHD typically begins 10 to 12 days after transfusion and is characterized by fever, skin rash, diarrhea, hepatitis, and marrow aplasia. TA-GVHD is fatal in most cases, usually because of host marrow failure resulting in overwhelming infection or bleeding. TA-GVHD can be prevented by gamma irradiation of cellular blood components, which render donor lymphocytes incapable of proliferating.[45] To prevent TA-GVHD in susceptible patients, blood and cellular components should be irradiated with at least 2500 cGy. In addition, all HLA-matched components, and all cellular components from blood relatives should be irradiated, regardless of patient diagnosis.

Immune Modulation

Immunomodulation refers to alterations in the recipient immune system as a result of transfusion. In some cases the immunologic effects are beneficial such as in prolongation of renal allograft survival or prevention of spontaneous abortion. There are also data, however, suggesting that the immunologic effects of transfusion may be deleterious in other clinical settings. These include an increased risk of tumor recurrence and postoperative bacterial infection. The relationship between blood transfusion and these clinical consequences are unproven and are the subject of ongoing research efforts.[46]

Hemosiderosis

One mL of red cells contains 1 mg of iron. Therefore, a unit of RBCs may contain 150 to 250 mg of iron. In individuals with chronic anemia, the continued need for red cell transfusion results in the accumulation of iron, which can eventually produce organ damage, particularly in the heart, liver, and pancreatic islets. There is no physiologic mechanism for excretion of excess iron. The parenteral iron chelator deferoxamine can prevent the complications of iron overload in patients receiving chronic red cell transfusion therapy.[47] Red cell exchange by apheresis has also been used to limit iron accumulation in patients with sickle cell disease who require repeated transfusions.

Air Embolism

Air embolism is rarely a problem with conventional transfusion techniques, but it may occur with the use of blood pumps and apheresis machines. Intraoperative infusion devices can infuse as much as 200 mL of air in 4 seconds. The frequency of fatal air embolism after readministration of recovered blood is 1:30,000 to 1:38,000.[48] Air embolism produces acute cardiopulmonary insufficiency as the air tends to migrate to the right ventricle, where it produces outlet obstruction. Acute cyanosis, pain, cough, arrythmia, shock, and cardiac arrest may result. Immediate treatment includes placing the patient head down on the left side in an attempt to dislodge the air bubble from the pulmonary valve.

Transfusion-Transmitted Diseases

Allogeneic blood donations are tested for hepatitis B surface antigen (HBsAg), antibody to hepatitis B core antigen (anti-HBc), antibody to hepatitis C (anti-HCV), antibody to human immunodeficiency virus, types 1/2 (anti-HIV-1/2), HIV p24 antigen, antibody to human T-cell lymphotropic virus, types I and II (anti-HTLV-I/II), a serologic test for syphilis, and nucleic acid testing (NAT) for HCV and HIV. Despite extensive donor screening and testing, infections can still be transmitted by blood transfusion. Most transmissions of hepatitis or HIV today occur from donors in the "window period" between infection and appearance of detectable antibody or virus. All cases of suspected posttransfusion infection should be reported to the blood bank, to identify infectious donors and prevent further transmissions.

Hepatitis

Hepatitis C virus (HCV) accounts for the majority of post-transfusion hepatitis. Transfusion accounts for 7% of chronic HCV infections today, mostly acquired before the implementation of serologic screening. Less than 20% of acute infections are symptomatic, and 85% of infections become chronic, which is usually asymptomatic. Among chronic carriers of HCV, cirrhosis occurs in 20% to 50% within 20 years and hepatocellular carcinoma in 15% to 20% by 30 years. In addition, chronic infection may lead to cryoglobulinemia and vasculitis. In contrast to HCV, acute hepatitis B virus (HBV) infection is symptomatic in 30% to 50% of adults, but less than 10% in children less than 5 years old. Chronic infection occurs in 2% to 10% of adults, but 30% to 90% of children less than 5 years old. Premature death from cirrhosis or hepatocellular carcinoma occurs in 15% to 25% of chronic carriers. Recent estimates of the window period for HBV and HCV are 60 to 150 days and 16 to 32 days respectively.[49] Estimates of the per unit risk of transfusion transmitted hepatitis are 1:137,00 for HBV and less than 1:1,00,000 for HCV.[49] Hepatitis A transmission has occurred with plasma derivatives, but is not a substantial risk for blood components. Hepatitis G virus may be transmitted by transfusion but does not appear to be associated with disease.

HIV

Transfusion-transmitted HIV has markedly declined since the implementation of antibody testing in 1985. The clinical manifestations of transfusion-transmitted HIV infection are similar to those of infections acquired through other routes. The rapidity with which the recipient progresses to AIDS is independent of status of the donor. Although the current transmission rate by transfusion is very low, new cases continue to be discovered due to past transfusions, usually through the look-back process of identifying recipients of blood from a donor subsequently diagnosed with HIV. Current donor screening tests are insensitive for group O HIV; however, this virus is very rare in the United States. The current estimated window period for HIV is 12 to 13 days. The per unit risk of HIV transmission is estimated to be 1:1,930,000, although it is difficult to be precise with such a low incidence.[49]

Other Viruses

Cytomegalovirus (CMV) infection is a major concern in immuno-suppressed recipients. Latent CMV infection is common among blood donors. CMV DNA can be found in leukocytes of many donors with antibody and some seronegative donors.[50] Transmission of CMV can be significantly reduced by either seronegative or leukocyte-reduced blood components, with equivalent efficacy.[51] Human T-cell lymphotrophic viruses are retroviruses unrelated to HIV. They are causally associated with adult T-cell lymphoma/leukemia (ATL) and peripheral neuropathy (HTLV-associated myelopathy, HAM). HTLV-I/II infections are rare in the United States. Because these viruses are strongly associated with white cells, leukocyte reduction may reduce transmission by transfusion. Parvovirus B19 causes erythema infectiosum in childhood. This virus can infect red cell precursors in marrow, and in patients with accelerated hematopoiesis can cause hypoplastic or aplastic anemia. Parvovirus can cause aplastic crisis in sickle cell disease, non-immune hydrops if acquired in pregnancy, and marrow transplant failure. Parvovirus B19 is common in the general population and can be found in high concentration in donor plasma.[52] Transmission by blood transfusion occurs, but seldom causes significant disease.[53] Epstein-Barr virus, human herpesvirus 8, and TT virus are transmissible by transfusion, but do appear to be of clinical significance in most transfusion recipients.

Parasites

Transfusion-transmitted malaria is uncommon in the United States, but does occur.[54] The most frequently implicated species is *Plasmodium falciparum*. The mortality rate of transfusion-transmitted malaria is 10%. Exclusion of high-risk donors is the most effective preventive measure. Transfusion-transmitted babesiosis has occurred in the United States. The parasitic reservoir is widely distributed in North America. Current serologic tests are inadequate for blood donor screening. Transfusion transmission of *Trypanosoma cruzi*, the cause of Chagas' disease, is a significant problem in areas of the world where the causative agent is endemic and has occurred in the United States. Serologic screening for *T. cruzi* infection may be effective where there is a high proportion of donors who emigrated from such areas.

Prions

Creutzfeldt-Jakob disease (CJD) is an illness caused by proteinaceous particles known as prions. Variant CJD (vCJD) differs from classical CJD in lack of affected family members, younger age of onset, more rapid progression, and association with consumption of certain animal products. No cases of CJD or vCJD transmission by blood transfusion have yet been reported. However, experimental models and theoretical considerations suggest that transmission by blood components is possible.[55,56] B cells and dendritic cells have been suggested to play a crucial role in the development of spongiform encephalopathy, which has led to the adoption of leukocyte reduction to minimize the risk of transfusion transmitted vCJD.[57,58] However, there are no data that universal leukocyte reduction will be efficacious in preventing spread of vCJD by transfused blood. At present there is no practical donor screening test for the abnormal isoform of the prion protein, although progress toward test development is being made.[59] Current strategies for reducing the theoretical risk of prion transmission include deferring donors with a family history of CJD, exposure to certain know risk factors, or residence in regions where vCJD is endemic.

References

1. Davenport RD. Hemolytic transfusion reactions. In: Popovsky MA, ed. Transfusion reactions, 2nd ed. Bethesda, MD: AABB Press, 2001:1-64.
2. Rother K, Till GO, eds. The complement system, 2nd ed. Berlin: Springer-Verlag, 1998.

3. Rodeberg DA, Chaet MS, Bass RC, et al. Nitric oxide: An overview. Am J Surg 1995;170:292-303.

4. Davenport RD. Inflammatory cytokines in hemolytic transfusion reactions. In: Davenport RD, Snyder EL, eds. Cytokines in transfusion medicine: A primer. Bethesda, MD: AABB Press, 1997:85-97.

5. Butler J, Parker D, Pillai R, et al. Systemic release of neutrophil elastase and tumour necrosis factor alpha following ABO incompatible blood transfusion. Br J Haematol 1991;79:525-6.

6. Davenport RD, Burdick M, Moore SA, Kunkel SL. Cytokine production in IgG mediated red cell incompatibility. Transfusion 1993;33:19-24.

7. Pierce RN, Reich LM, Mayer K. Hemolysis following platelet transfusions from ABO-incompatible donors. Transfusion 1985;25:60-2.

8. Kim HC, Park CL, Cowan JH, et al. Massive intravascular hemolysis associated with intravenous immunoglobulin in bone marrow transplant recipients. Am J Pediatr Hematol Oncol 1988;10:69-74.

9. Mair B, Benson K. Evaluation of changes in hemoglobin levels associated with ABO-incompatible plasma in apheresis platelets. Transfusion 1998;38:51-5.

10. Petz LD, Calhoun L, Shulman IA, et al. The sickle cell hemolytic transfusion reaction syndrome. Transfusion 1997;37:382-92.

11. King KE, Shirey RS, Lankiewicz MW, et al. Delayed hemolytic transfusion reactions in sickle cell disease: Simultaneous destruction of recipients' red cells. Transfusion 1997;37:376-81.

12. Arndt PA, Leger RM, Garratty G. Serology of antibodies to second- and third-generation cephalosporins associated with immune hemolytic anemia and/or positive direct antiglobulin tests Transfusion 1999;39:1239-46.

13. Perkins HA, Payne R, Ferguson J, Wood M. Non-hemolytic febrile transfusion reactions. Quantitative effects of blood components with emphasis on isoantigenic incompatibility of leukocytes. Vox Sang 1966;11:578-99.

14. Heddle NM, Kelton JG. Febrile nonhemolytic transfusion reactions. In: Popovsky MA, ed. Transfusion reactions, 2nd ed. Bethesda, MD: AABB Press, 2001:45-82.

15. Mangano MM, Chambers LA, Kruskall MS. Limited efficacy of leukopoor platelets for prevention of febrile transfusion reactions. Am J Clin Pathol 1991;95:733-8.

16. Lane TA, Anderson KC, Goodnough LT, et al. Leukocyte reduction in blood component therapy. Ann Intern Med 1992;117:151-62.

17. Heddle NM, Klama L, Singer J, et al. The role of the plasma from platelet concentrates in transfusion reactions. N Engl J Med 1994;331:625-8.

18. Aye MT, Palmer DS, Giulivi A, et al. Effects of filtration of platelet concentrates on the accumulation of cytokines and platelet release factors during storage. Transfusion 1995;35:117-24.

19. Uhlmann EJ, Isgriggs E, Wallhermfechtel M, Goodnough LT. Prestorage universal WBC reduction of RBC units does not affect the incidence of transfusion reactions. Transfusion 2001; 41:997-1000.

20. Tanz WS, King KE, Ness PM. Reevaluation of transfusion reaction rates associated with leukocyte-reduced red blood cells (abstract). Transfusion 2001; 41:7S.

21. Phipps RP, Kaufman J, Blumberg N. Platelet derived CD154 (CD40 ligand) and febrile responses to transfusion. Lancet 2001;357:2023-4.

22. Vyas GN, Perkins HA, Fudenberg HH. Anaphylactoid transfusion reactions associated with anti-IgA. Lancet 1968;ii:312-5.

23. Westhoff CM, Sipherd BD, Wylie DE, Toalson LD. Severe anaphylactic reaction following transfusion of platelets to a patient with anti-Ch. Transfusion 1992; 32:576-9.

24. Koda Y, Watanabe Y, Soejima M et al. Simple PCR detection of haptoglobin gene deletion in anhaptoglobinemic patients with antihaptoglobin antibody that causes anaphylactic transfusion reactions. Blood 2000; 95:1138-43.

25. Davenport RD, Burnie KL, Barr RM. Transfusion management of patients with IgA deficiency and anti-IgA during liver transplantation. Vox Sang 1992; 63:247-50.

26. Popovsky MA, Moore SB. Diagnostic and pathogenic considerations in transfusion-related acute lung injury. Transfusion 1985;25:573-7.

27. Popovsky MA, Davenport RD. Transfusion-related acute lung injury: Femme fatale? Transfusion 2001;41:312-5.

28. Silliman CC, Paterson AJ, Dickey WO, et al. The association of biologically active lipids with the development of transfusion-related acute lung injury: A retrospective study. Transfusion 1997;37:719-26.

29. Shiba M, Tadokoro K, Sawanobori M, et al. Activation of the contact system by filtration of platelet concentrates with a negatively charged white cell removal filter and measurement of venous blood bradykinin level in patients who received filtered platelets. Transfusion 1997;37:457-62.

30. Hild M, Soderstrom T, Egberg N, et al. Kinetics of bradykinin levels during and after leucocyte filtration of platelet concentrates. Vox Sang 1998;75:18-25.

31. Mair B, Leparc GF. Hypotensive reactions associated with platelet transfusions and angiotensin-converting enzyme inhibitors. Vox Sang 1998;74:27-30.

32. De Korte D, Marcelis JH, Soeterboek AM. Determination of the degree of bacterial contamination of whole-blood collections using an automated microbe-detection system. Transfusion 2001;41:815-8.

33. Perez P, Salmi LR, Folléa G, et al. Determinants of transfusion-associated bacterial contamination: results of the French BACTHEM Case-Control Study. Transfusion 2001;41:862-72.

34. Dzik WH, Kirkley SA. Citrate toxicity during massive blood transfusion. Transfus Med Rev 1988;2:76-94.

35. Driscoll DF, Bistrian BR, Jenkins RL, et al. Development of metabolic alkalosis after massive transfusion during orthopedic liver transplantation. Crit Care Med 1987;15:905-8.

36. Lostumbo MM, Holland PV, Schmidt PJ. Isoimmunization after multiple transfusions. N Engl J Med 1966;275:141-4.

37. Kohan AI, Niborski RC, Rey JA, et al. High-dose intravenous immunoglobulin in non-ABO transfusion incompatibility. Vox Sang 1994; 67:195-8.

38. Mueller-Eckhardt CH. Post-transfusion purpura. Br J Haematol 1986;64:419.

39. Laursen B, Morling N, Rosenkvist J, et al. Post-transfusion purpura treated with plasma exchange by Haemonetics cell separator. Acta Med Scand 1978;203:539-43.

40. Linden JV, Pisciotto PT. Transfusion-associated graft-versus-host disease and blood irradiation. Transfus Med Rev 1992;6:116-23.

41. Holland PV. Prevention of transfusion-associated graft-vs-host disease. Arch Pathol Lab Med 1989;113:285-91.

42. Thaler M, Shamiss A, Orgad S, et al. The role of blood from HLA homozygous donors in fatal transfusion-associated graft-versus-host disease after open heart surgery. N Engl J Med 1989;321:25-8.

43. Shivdasani RA, Haluska FG, Dock NL, et al. Graft-versus-host disease associated with transfusion of blood from unrelated HLA-homozygous donors. N Engl J Med 1993;328:766-70.

44. Krenger W, Ferrara JLM. Dysregulation of cytokines during graft-versus-host disease. J Hematother 1996;5:3-14.

45. Moroff G, Luban NLC. The irradiation of blood and blood components to prevent graft-versus-host disease: Technical issues and guidelines. Transfus Med Rev 1997;11: 15-26.

46. Vamvakas EC, Dzik WH, Blajchman MA. Deleterious effects of transfusion-associated immunomodulation: Appraisal of the evidence and recommendations for prevention. In: Vamvakas EC, Blajchman MA, eds. Immunomodulatory effects of blood transfusion. Besthesda, MD: AABB Press,1999:256-86.

47. Marcus CS, Huehns ER. Transfusional iron overload. Clin Lab Haematol 1985;7:195-212.

48. Linden, J, Kaplan H, Murphy MT. Fatal air embolism due to perioperative blood recovery. Anesth Analg 1997;84: 422-6.

49. Busch MP. Closing the windows on viral transmission by blood transfusion. In: Stramer SL, ed. Blood safety in the new millennium. Besthesda, MD: American Association of Blood Banks, 2001:33-54.

50. Larsson S, Soderberg-Naucler C, Wang FZ, Moller E. Cytomegalovirus DNA can be detected in peripheral blood mononuclear cells from all seropositive and most sero-negative healthy blood donors over time. Transfusion 1998;38:271-8.

51. Bowden RA, Slichter SJ, Sayers M, et al. A comparison of filtered leukocyte-reduced and cytomegalovirus (CMV) seronegative blood products for the prevention of transfusion-associated CMV infection after marrow transplantation. Blood 1995;86:3598-603.

52. Weimer T, Streichert S, Watson C, Gröner A. High-titer screening PCR: a successful strategy for reducing the parvovirus B19 load in plasma pools for fractionation. Transfusion 2001;41:1500-4.

53. Koenigbauer UF, Eastland T, Day JW. Clinical illness due to parvovirus B19 infection after infusion of solvent/detergent-treated pooled plasma. Transfusion 2000;40:1203-6.

54. Mungai M, Tegtmeier G, Chamberland M, Parise M. Transfusion-transmitted malaria in the United States from 1963 through 1999. N Engl J Med 2001;344:1973-8.

55. Brown P, Rohwer RG, Dunstan BC, et al. The distribution of infectivity in blood components and plasma derivatives in experimental models of transmissible spongiform encephalopathy. Transfusion 1998;38:810-6.

56. Houston F, Foster JD, Chong A, et al. Transmission of BSE by blood transfusion in sheep. Lancet 2000;356:999-1000.

57. Klein MA, Frigg R, Flechsig E, et al. A crucial role for B cells in neuroinvasive scrapie. Nature 1997;390:687-90.

58. Klein MA, Frigg R, Raeber AJ, et al. PrP expression in B lymphocytes is not required for prion neuroinvasion. Nat Med 1998;4:1429-33.

59. MacGregor I. Prion protein and developments in its detection. Transfus Med 2001;11:3-14.

HEMATOPOIETIC PROGENITOR CELLS

Concept of Hematopoietic Therapy

Hematopoietic progenitor cells (HPCs) may be obtained from the patient (autologous), from an identical twin (syngeneic), or from a related or unrelated individual (allogeneic). Allogeneic HPCs are used therapeutically for the treatment of hematologic malignancies, marrow failure, immunodeficiency syndromes, and inborn errors of metabolism. Autologous HPC therapy is used in the treatment of hematologic and other maligancies and nonmalignant conditions (ie, autoimmune disorders). In autologous transplantation, HPCs are primarily used for hematopoietic "rescue" in patients who have received myeloablative therapy (ie, chemotherapy, radiation). In allogeneic HPC transplantation there is an additional benefit; T cells in the graft attack residual tumor cells in what has been called the graft-vs-leukemia effect. These T cells also mediate the primary complication of allogeneic HPC therapy, graft-vs-host disease (GVHD), which results in the higher transplant-related morbidity and mortality compared with autologous HPC therapy. HPCs are also used to reconstitute marrow function in marrow failure syndromes such as aplastic anemia, or immune function in immunodeficiency states. In the near future, HPCs could serve as a vehicle for gene therapy such as in the treatment of severe combined immunodeficiency. Recent breakthrough discoveries of the plasticity of adult stem cells has shown that HPCs can potentially be used to generate a variety of nonhematopoietic tissue cell types, such as heart, lung, liver, muscle, brain, and etc.[1] Advances in the collection and processing of HPCs, development of the capability to expand hematopoietic cells, and the promise of solid organ repair and gene therapy are likely to increase the indications for HPC therapy.

Marrow

Description of Component

Marrow may be obtained from autologous, syngeneic, or allogeneic donors. It is harvested from hematopoietically active, readily accessible skeletal sites, usually the iliac crests in adults. Harvesting is performed in the operating room under general, spinal, or epidural anesthesia, and is accomplished by multiple punctures and aspirations of the iliac crest. Marrow is aspirated into citrate or heparin anticoagulant and filtered (200- to 300-micron pore size) to remove clots, bone fragments, and fat. About 0.5-1.5 L of marrow (10 to 15 mL/kg donor weight) is harvested from adults, containing approximately 1.0 to 1.5×10^{10} nucleated cells, exclusive of nucleated red cells.[2] It is variably diluted with peripheral blood, depending on the harvesting procedure. Autologous marrow may also contain malignant cells if they are present in the patient's marrow. Marrow may be processed in the laboratory in order to 1) prevent hemolysis by removal of donor plasma antibodies incompatible with recipient red cells, or by removal of donor red cells incompatible with recipient plasma antibodies; 2) diminish or eliminate autologous malignant cells that might contribute to disease relapse; 3) diminish the severity of GVHD by reducing the content of donor T cells; or 4) accomplish all of the above and reduce overall volume by selection and concentration of early HPCs (eg, cells that carry the CD34 antigen). Consequently, the final product may have a variable volume, hematocrit, and cell count. Marrow may be stored frozen in cryopreservative containing dimethylsulfoxide (DMSO). Cryopreserved marrow must be infused as soon as possible after thawing (30 minutes to 1 hour) to maintain cell viability. Fresh noncryopreserved marrow may be stored at 4 to 6 C or at 20 to 24 C for up to 24 hours before infusion and still maintain good cell viability.

Indications

Allogeneic and syngeneic marrow are intended to provide permanent lymphohematopoietic engraftment after transplantation.[3] Potential allogeneic marrow donors must be tissue-matched carefully with the recipient to ensure engraftment and diminish the risk of GVHD. Red cell compatibility testing between donor and recipient must be performed to assess the need for additional marrow processing to prevent hemolysis of donor or recipient red cells.

Contraindications and Precautions

Marrow transplantation carries a high risk of recipient mortality and is performed only in facilities with a specially trained transplant team. Donor risks include those associated with general anesthesia and local discomfort. If needed, blood transfusion to replace blood lost by the donor during marrow harvesting (see above) should also be considered a risk. Consequently, preoperative autologous blood donation may be employed. Any allogeneic blood given to the marrow donor during the harvesting procedure should be irradiated to prevent transfusion-associated GVHD in the marrow recipient. Recipient risks inherent in marrow transplantation include those associated with treatment (conditioning) regimen toxicity (eg, veno-occlusive disease of the liver, interstitial pulmonary disease), prolonged cytopenia (eg, infections, hemorrhage), immune suppression [eg, reactivation of cytomegalovirus (CMV) infection], and disease relapse. Risks associated with the transplant product include graft rejection, GVHD, hemolysis, or delayed engraftment due to donor-recipient red cell incompatibility, microbial contamination, transmission of viral infection, and acute reactions associated with infusion of DMSO.

Common side effects of DMSO include an unpleasant taste or smell, nausea, vomiting, diarrhea, chills, and hypertension. Anaphylactoid reactions (flushing, hypotension, bronchospasm, pulmonary edema) may also occur due to release of bradykinin and histamine. Cardiovascular effects of DMSO such as cardiac arrhythmias and neurologic symptoms have rarely been observed.[4]

Dose and Administration

The minimal effective dose of HPCs has not been clearly established. However, centers are increasingly using the measurement of CD34-positive cells (or CD34 subsets) to assess cell dose. The target dose recommended by the National Marrow Donor Program (NMDP) is 2 to 4×10^8 nucleated cells/kg recipient body weight.[4] It is common practice to administer marrow without a standard blood filter, and leukocyte-reduction filters must *never* be used during marrow infusion because they may remove hematopoietic cells. Likewise, marrow should *never* be irradiated because irradiation will prevent HPCs from engrafting. The optimal storage temperature (4 C vs room temperature) and upper limit of shelf life have not been defined, but it has been recommended that marrow should be infused as soon as practicable after processing, and preferably within 24 hours.[5] Marrow shipped overnight at room temperature has successfully engrafted patients treated through the NMDP. When cryopreserved, marrow is generally thawed at the bedside at 37 to 40 C and infused immediately without filtration, preferably through a central venous catheter. Unlike blood components, all marrow for transplantation represents a sometimes irreplaceable life-sparing biologic product that is specifically designated for a given patient. Consequently, extra effort must be made to ensure that the marrow is properly handled, that cell viability is maintained during storage and transport, and that the recipient receives the product in a timely manner.

Peripheral Blood Progenitor Cells

Description of Component

Very small numbers of HPCs are found in the peripheral blood of normal individuals. The number of circulating peripheral blood progenitor cells (PBPCs) may be increased (or "mobilized" from the marrow) up to 100-fold or higher by administration of hematopoietic growth factors such as granulocyte colony-stimulating factor (G-CSF) and granulocyte-macrophage colony-stimulating factor (GM-CSF) (see Hematopoietic Growth Factors). These agents are used alone for allogeneic donors. However, they are often used in conjunction with the rebound of the leukocyte count from chemotherapy-induced cytopenia for autologous transplant patients.[6] Mobilized PBPCs are collected by one or more leukapheresis procedures during which two to three blood volumes (10 to 20 L) are processed,[4] typically yielding 1 to 8 $\times 10^{10}$ leukocytes, containing 0.1% to 5% of CD34-positive leukocytes. The adequacy of PBPC collection is increasingly based on the number of cells bearing the CD34 antigen. These cells represent early hematopoietic progenitors, and a small subpopulation is thought to be true multipotent hematopoietic stem cells. PBPCs may be stored frozen in a cryopreservative containing DMSO. After thawing, they must be infused as soon as possible to maintain viability (15 to 30 minutes).

Indications

PBPCs may be used alone or as a supplement to marrow infusion for autologous or allogeneic[7] transplantation. Potential advantages in the use of mobilized PBPCs rather than marrow collection include a diminished duration of severe cytopenia after transplant (8 to 10 days for neutrophil engraftment and 10 to 12 days for platelet engraftment), avoidance of donor hospitalization, avoidance of general anesthesia during collection, and reduced incidence of tumor cell contamination in autologous transplantation.[8] Potential disadvantages of PBPCs include some difficulties in determining the optimal timing of leukapheresis, vascular access problems, and the need to perform multiple leukapheresis procedures in order to collect sufficient numbers of progenitor cells, especially in poorly mobilized patients. Generally, PBPC collection can start with a peripheral blood CD34 count of as low as 5 cells/μL, but if possible, it should start with a CD34 count of at least 10 to 20 cells/μL. Studies show that sufficient numbers of progenitor cells to perform syngeneic and allogeneic marrow transplants,[7,9,10] can

141

be mobilized into the peripheral blood of normal donors with use of G-CSF and/or GM-CSF alone.

Contraindications and Precautions

Side effects and hazards are similar to those for marrow. Infusion of multiple collections from poorly mobilized patients often results in an increased incidence and severity of DMSO toxicity due to large amounts of DMSO exposure. Because DMSO toxicity is dose-dependent, it is recommended that the maximal amounts of DMSO infused should not exceed 1 mg/kg per session.[4]

Dose and Administration

A therapeutic dose of PBPCs has not been defined. Doses of 6 × 10^8 mononuclear cells (MNCs)/kg recipient body weight have been recommended; however, the number of MNCs correlates poorly with engraftment, and most centers now recommend a target dose of either >3 to 5 × 10^5 mobilized granulocyte/macrophage colony-forming units (CFU-GM) per kg, or >1 to 6 × 10^6 CD34-positive cells per kg to ensure rapid hematopoietic engraftment.[11-13] As with marrow, the use of leukocyte-reduction filters and irradiation are contraindicated. The optimal storage temperature and upper limit of shelf life have not been defined. PBPCs can be frozen in 10% DMSO in a controlled rate freezer and store in vapor phase of liquid nitrogen. PBPCs can also be frozen in a mechanical freezer at <–80 C. The frozen PBPC product should be infused as soon as practical after thawing or if kept refrigerated as soon as possible after processing.

Cord Blood Products

Cord blood obtained from a delivered placenta is known to be rich in early and committed progenitor cells.[14] Since the first cord blood transplant was reported in 1989 for Fanconi anemia,[15] more than 2000 patients have been transplanted with cord blood for a variety of malignant and nonmalignant conditions.[16] The great majority of cord blood transplants have been from unrelated donors and approximately 10% to 15% have been from sibling donors.[17] Cord blood is collected from the placenta at the time of delivery using either an open or closed system. The volume is typically 80 to 100 mL (range 40 to 240 mL) with a mean nucleated cell content of $1.4 \times 10^9 \pm 1.0 \times 10^9$.[18] The CD34 content has been reported to be $1.4 \times 10^5 \pm 1.8 \times 10^5$ cells/kg (0.01% to 1.0% of nucleated cells).[19] Clinical studies have reported successful engraftment in children[19,20] with a higher risk of graft failure in patients weighing more than 45 kg.[20] The median time to neutrophil engraftment (500/µL) is 30 days and platelet engraftment (20,000/µL) is 56 days.[20] While neutrophil engraftment is similar to that observed after allogeneic marrow transplantation, platelet engraftment appears to be delayed.[17] Currently it is recommended to infuse at least 3×10^7 total nucleated cells/kg patient weight, with a minimal safety dose of 1.5×10^7 total nucleated cells/kg.[16] In addition to HLA-matched cord blood transplants, which are associated with high relapse rate, 5/6 HLA-matched cord blood transplants can also be carried out sucessfully, if CD34 count is high.[21] Clinical studies have also suggested that unrelated marrow transplants are associated with a lower risk of GVHD compared with unrelated marrow transplants in children.[19,20]

The advantages of cord blood as a source of hematopoietic cells for transplantation include: no risk to donor, lower risk of viral infection, potential availability of cord blood from ethnic minorities under-represented in the NMDP and other donor registries, more rapid availability of cord blood cells for transplantation, and possibly lower risk of GVHD. Disadvantages of cord blood include ethical and informed consent issues,[22] and concerns about engraftment in adults as a result of the limited number of nucleated cells in cord blood. Techniques for ex-vivo expansion and pooling of cord blood HPCs are currently under investigation and may eventually allow routine transplantation in adults.[23,24] Future clinical studies will need to address additional issues such as the minimum number of cells needed for engraftment in adults, the risks of GVHD in HLA-mismatched unrelated cord blood transplants, relapse rates, the graft-vs-leukemia effect, the potential for gene therapy with autologous cord blood HPCs, immunologic reconstitution, and generation of nonhematopoietic tissue cell types.[17]

Donor Leukocyte Infusion

Donor leukocyte infusion (DLI) has been increasingly used after allogeneic transplantation. The indications include treatment of relapsed chronic myelogenous leukemia and less frequently acute myelogenous leukemia or acute lymphocytic leukemia; DLI works via a graft-vs-leukemia effect. DLI is also used for treatment of posttransplantation Epstein-Barr virus (EBV) or CMV infection by restoring cell-mediated immunity in the recipient. A typical DLI dose is 1×10^8 CD3+/kg recipient body weight for treatment of relapsed leukemia, which can be collected by 1 or 2 apheresis procedures. A smaller dose is required for treatment of CMV or EBV infection. Complications of DLI include GVHD and pancytopenia.[4]

Hematopoietic Growth Factors

Erythropoietin

Erythropoietin (EPO) is a glycoprotein growth factor that stimulates the division and differentiation of committed red cell precursors in the marrow. EPO prepared by recombinant DNA technology (rHuEPO) has been approved for use in anemic patients with chronic renal failure (serum creatinine >1.8 mg/dL) to stimulate red cell production and reduce the need for RBC transfusions.[25,26] The approved dose is 50 to 100 U/kg body weight intravenously or subcutaneously 1 to 3 times per week. This dose is reduced when the hematocrit reaches 30% to 34%. rHuEPO has also been approved to treat anemia in zidovudine-treated HIV-infected patients with endogenous EPO levels <500 mU/mL[27] and in cancer patients on chemotherapy.[28] One study has shown that there may be a quality of life benefit in chemotherapy patients treated with rHuEPO.[29] rHuEPO has demonstrated some efficacy in other investigational settings including the anemia of chronic disease, the anemia of prematurity, marrow transplantation, and autologous blood donation.[26] rHuEPO also has been shown to be beneficial in a subset of patients with myelodysplastic syndrome and aplastic anemia but is of questionable benefit in sickle cell disease and the setting of surgical blood loss.[26] The major adverse effects in patients with chronic renal failure treated with rHuEPO have been the development or exacerbation of hypertension, headache, and a concern about an increased incidence of thrombotic episodes. A recent publication describes red cell aplasia due to development of EPO antibodies in chronic renal failure patients.[30] Some preparations of rHuEPO use human albumin as a stabilizer. Patients receiving rHuEPO may require iron supplementation to ensure adequate iron stores for erythropoiesis.

Colony-Stimulating Factors

The cloning of genes encoding the human growth factors has led to clinical trials of several myeloid colony-stimulating factors.[26,31] These factors are used alone or in combination to stimulate the proliferation and differentiation of hematopoietic progenitors. They appear to reduce the period of neutropenia after cytotoxic chemotherapy administration and hematopoietic transplantation. Two of these factors have been approved for clinical use. G-CSF exerts its primary in-vivo effects on late progenitors known as granulocyte colony-forming units (CFU-G). When the appropriate progenitors capable of responding to the exogenously administered cytokine are present, the circulating leukocyte count rapidly increases. This reflects both a release of mature neutrophils from the storage pool and a decrease in the cycling time for mature progenitors. G-CSF decreases the duration of neutropenia and the incidence of infection in patients receiving myelosuppressive chemotherapy. G-CSF has also been used successfully in certain investigational settings including congenital agranulocytosis, acute leukemia, myelodysplastic syndrome, aplastic anemia in children, and the mobilization of PBPCs for autologous or allogeneic marrow transplantation.[10,32] The combination of G-CSF and dexamethasone given the evening before granulocytapheresis (normal donors) may also greatly enhance the yield of granulocytes.[33] This may expand the therapeutic use of these cells.[34] G-CSF not only exerts its effects on the late CFU-GM, but it also works either directly or synergistically with other hematopoietic growth factors to stimulate progenitor cell growth. Like G-CSF, GM-CSF enhances the function of mature myeloid cells lines. It has been used to accelerate myeloid recovery in patients undergoing marrow transplantation and chemotherapy.[31,35] Guidelines have been published regarding the use of GM-CSF and G-CSF in oncology patients.[36] These growth factors have also been used in the treatment of myelodysplastic syndrome and leukopenia in AIDS.[10] Side effects seen with G-CSF and GM-CSF include bone pain, myalgias, anorexia, and fever. When GM-CSF is used at high doses (eg, >15 mg/kg), fluid retention, pericarditis, pleural effusions, and serositis have occurred. A polyethylene glycol derivative preparation of G-CSF (Neulasta or pegfilgrastim) has recently been licensed by the Food and Drug Administration (FDA).

Several new growth factors with hematopoietic activity include NESP (novel erythropoiesis stimulating protein), c-kit ligand, Flt3 ligand, and interleukin-11.[37-39] NESP (Aranesp or darbepoetin alfa), an erythropoietin analogue, has a longer half-life and increased activity compared with EPO. In treating anemia and chronic renal insufficiency, NESP given once weekly, intravenously or subcutaneously, has been shown to be as effective as EPO given twice weekly.[37,38] The clinical efficacy of interleukin-11 (currently licensed by the FDA) in promoting megakarycytopoiesis appears to be limited.[40] A truncated, polyethylene glycol derivative preparation of thrombopoietin (megakaryocyte growth and development factor) has been studied for its ability to increase circulating platelet counts in thrombocytopenic patients and plateletpheresis donors.[41,42] However, the development of neutralizing antibodies and iatrogenic thrombocytopenia has resulted in the closure of clinical trials.[43] Other preparations of this growth factor with thrombopoietic activity are under investigation.

Transfusion Therapy in HPC Transplantation

Prior to transplantation, cellular blood components should be leukocyte-reduced to prevent alloimmunization and, in susceptible hosts, CMV transmission.[44] The development of alloimmunization to histocompatibility antigens poses an increased risk for subsequent graft rejection, especially for patients with aplastic anemia.[45,46] Therefore, blood component exposure should be minimized and transfusions from potential progenitor cell donors should be particularly avoided. After transplantation, patients typically experience 2 or more weeks of marrow aplasia, during which extensive red cell and platelet support is required. The use of PBPCs and hematopoietic growth factors have shortened this interval and diminished the requirement for transfusion support. In contrast, cord blood transplants are frequently associated with a prolonged need for platelet support.[20,21] If ABO differences between donor and recipient exist, the patient's blood group will change, and careful planning is required. Such ABO mismatches can be major (eg, transplant from a type A donor to an O patient), or minor (eg, transplant from a type O donor to an A patient). In major mismatches, the recipient is at risk for severe intravascular hemolysis of red cells in the marrow graft; this can be prevented by erythrocyte depletion of the graft before transplant.[47] In PBPC transplants, the red cell content is generally so low (<50 mL) that red cell depletion is not required. Additional complications include delayed red cell engraftment and late hemolysis of engrafted donor red cells at 40 to 60 days after transplantation due to residual host anti-A or -B.[48,49] Similar problems may be encountered if the recipient has a clinically relevant alloantibody to an antigen expressed on the donor's red cells. The immediate hazards of minor mismatches can be avoided by depleting the graft of incompatible plasma.[47] However, engrafted donor lymphocytes may produce antibodies against recipient red cell antigens, which can result in hemolysis of residual recipient red cells 1 to 3 weeks after transplantation. For these reasons, a blood bank consultation should be obtained for any patient receiving an ABO- or Rh-mismatched transplant, and both pre- and posttransplant transfusion therapy should be planned in close cooperation with the blood bank. A practical transfusion guideline for ABO- mismatched allogeneic transplantation is provided in Table 6.

All transplant recipients are profoundly immunosuppressed and thus at risk for fatal TA-GVHD after transfusions of cellular blood components. Consequently, all such transfusion units must be gamma irradiated (25 Gy or 2500 cGy) prior to use. Transplant recipients are also at risk for hematopoietic transplant-associated GVHD, which is caused by the engraftment of lymphocytes contained in the progenitor cell product. GVHD occurs commonly after allogeneic transplantation, and is generally treatable. The incidence of chronic, rather than acute, GVHD is greater after PBPC than marrow transplantation, presumably because of the higher content of T cells in PBPCs.[50,51] T-cell depletion, typically to <10^5 T cells/kg, has been employed to reduce the incidence of GVHD, but at the expense of increased graft failure, infection rate, and relapse. The progenitor cell product must *never* be irradiated, as this would prevent engraftment.

Cytomegalovirus infection develops frequently following HPC transplantation and may be associated with high morbidity.[47] The risk of infection is influenced most by the CMV serologic status of the recipient before transplantation.[52] Cellular blood component (or HPC) transfusions from CMV-seropositive donors to CMV-seronegative recipients may lead to seroconversion and symptomatic infection. Seropositive transplant recipients may experience reactivation of latent CMV infection regardless of donor serostatus. Although newer therapeutic advances (eg, gancyclovir) may reduce the incidence and severity of CMV infection, all CMV-seronegative transplant patients should receive cellular blood components that have been CMV screened or processed using a prestorage 3 to 4 log leukocyte reduction filter to reduce the risk of CMV transmission.[53] In contrast, CMV-positive transplant patients and those receiving transplants from CMV-positive donors have not been shown to benefit from the use of CMV-seronegative blood products.

Autologous marrow and PBPC transplantation have fewer transfusion-related hazards. The donor and recipient are by definition ABO- and HLA-identical. Although the degree of posttransplant immunosuppression is reduced, all cellular blood components (except the transplant itself) must nevertheless be ir-

Table 6. Transfusion Support for Patients Undergoing ABO-Mismatched Allogeneic HPC Transplantation

Recipient	Donor	Mismatch Type	Phase I — All Components	RBCs	Phase II — First Choice Platelets	Next Choice Platelets*	FFP	Phase III — All Components
A	O	Minor	Recipient	O	A	AB; B; O	A, AB	Donor
B	O	Minor	Recipient	O	B	AB; A; O	B, AB	Donor
AB	O	Minor	Recipient	O	AB	A; B; O	AB	Donor
AB	A	Minor	Recipient	A	AB	A; B; O	AB	Donor
AB	B	Minor	Recipient	B	AB	B; A; O	AB	Donor
O	A	Major	Recipient	O	A	AB; B; O	A, AB	Donor
O	B	Major	Recipient	O	B	AB; A; O	B, AB	Donor
O	AB	Major	Recipient	O	AB	A; B; O	AB	Donor
A	AB	Major	Recipient	A	AB	A; B; O	AB	Donor

(Continued)

149

Table 6. Transfusion Support for Patients Undergoing ABO-Mismatched Allogeneic HPC Transplantation (Continued)

Recipient	Donor	Mismatch Type	Phase I All Components	Phase II RBCs	Phase II First Choice Platelets	Phase II Next Choice Platelets*	Phase II FFP	Phase III All Components
B	AB	Major	Recipient	B	AB	B; A; O	AB	Donor
A	B	Minor & major	Recipient	O	AB	A; B; O	AB	Donor
B	A	Minor & major	Recipient	O	AB	B; A; O	AB	Donor

*Platelet concentrates should be selected in the order presented. Modified from Friedberg.[125]

Phase I = from the time when the patient/recipient is prepared for HPC transplantation.

Phase II = from the initiation of myeloablative therapy until:

 For RBC—DAT is negative and antidonor isohemagglutinins are no longer detectable (ie, the reverse typing is donor type)

 For FFPs—recipient's erythrocytes are no longer detectable (ie, the forward typing is consistent with donor's ABO group)

Phase III = after the forward and reverse typing of the patient are consistent with donor's ABO group.

Beginning from Phase I all cellular components should be irradiated and leukocyte reduced.

Used with permission from Brecher ME, ed. Technical manual, 14th ed. Bethesda, MD: American Association of Blood Banks, 2002:556.

radiated. CMV-seronegative patients should receive CMV-reduced-risk cellular components.

References

1. Krause DS, Theise ND, Collector MI, et al. Multi-organ, multi-lineage engraftment by a single bone marrow-derived stem cell. Cell 2000;105(3):369-77.
2. Treleaven JG, Mehta J. Bone marrow and peripheral blood stem cell harvesting. J Hematother 1992;1:215-23.
3. Armitage JO. Bone marrow transplantation. N Engl J Med 1994;330:827-38.
4. Snyder EL, Haley NR, eds. Hematopietic progenitor cells: A primer for medical professionals. Bethesda, MD: AABB Press, 2000.
5. National Marrow Donor Program Standards, 13th edition. Minneapolis, MN: National Marrow Donor Program, 1996.
6. To LB, Haylock DN, Simmons PJ, Juttner CA. The biology and clinical uses of blood stem cells. Blood 1997; 897:2233-58.
7. Bensinger WI, Weaver CH, Appelbaum FR, et al. Transplantation of allogeneic peripheral blood stem cells mobilized by recombinant human granulocyte colony-stimulating factor. Blood 1995;85:6:1655-8.
8. Juttner CA, Fibbe WE, Nemunaitis J, et al. Blood cell transplantation: Report from an international consensus meeting. Bone Marrow Transplant 1994;14:689-93.
9. Korbling M, Przepiorka D, Huh YO, et al. Allogeneic blood stem cell transplantation for refractory leukemia and lymphoma: Potential advantage of blood over marrow allografts. Blood 1995;85:1659-65.
10. Lane TA, Law P, Maruyama M, et al. Harvesting and enrichment of hematopoietic stem cells mobilized into the peripheral blood of normal donors by granulocyte-macrophage colony stimulating factor (GM-CSF) or G-CSF: Potential role in allogeneic marrow transplantation. Blood 1995;85:275-82.

11. Haas R, Mohle R, Fruhauf S, et al. Patient characteristics associated with successful mobilizing and autografting of peripheral blood progenitor cells in malignant lymphoma. Blood 1994;83:3787-94.

12. To LB. Assaying the CFU-GM in blood: Correlation between cell dose and haemopoietic reconstitution. Bone Marrow Transplant 1990;5(suppl 1):16-8.

13. Schwartzberg L, Birch R, Blanco R, et al. Rapid and sustained hematopoietic reconstitution by peripheral blood stem cell infusion alone following high-dose chemotherapy. Bone Marrow Transplant 1993;11:369-74.

14. Broxmeyer HE, Gluckman E, Auerbach AD, et al. Human umbilical cord blood: A clinically useful source of transplantable hematopoietic stem/progenitor cells. Int J Cell Cloning 1990;8:76.

15. Gluckman E, Broxmeyer HE, Auerbach AD, et al. Hematopoietic reconstitution in a patient with Fanconi anemia by means of umbilical-cord blood from an HLA- identical siblings. N Engl J Med 1989;321:1174.

16. Szczepiorkowski ZM, Snyder EL, eds. Current perspectives in cellular therapy 2002. Bethesda, MD: American Association of Blood Banks, 2001.

17. Cairo MS, Wagner JE. Placental and/or umbilical cord blood: An alternative source of hematopoietic stem cells for transplantation. Blood 1997;90:4665-78.

18. Wagner WE, Broxmeyer HE, Cooper S. Umbilical cord and placental blood hematopoietic stem cells: Collection, cryopreservation, and storage. J Hematother 1992;1:167-73.

19. Kurtzberg J, Laughlin M, Graham ML, et al. Placental blood as a source of hematopoietic stem cells for transplantation into unrelated recipients. N Engl J Med 1996;3:335:157-66.

20. Gluckman E, Rocha V, Boyer-Chammard A, et al. Outcome of cord-blood transplantation from related and unrelated donors. Eurocord Transplant Group and the European Blood and Marrow Transplantation Group. N Engl J Med 1997;337:373-81.

21. Rubinstein P, Carrier C, Scaradavou A, et al. Outcomes among 562 recipients of placental-blood transplants from unrelated donors. N Engl J Med 1998;339:1565-77.

22. Haley R, Harvath L, Sugarman J. Ethical issues in cord blood banking: Summary of a workshop. Transfusion 1998;38:867-73.

23. Ende N, Lu S, Alcid MG, et al. Pooled umbilical cord blood as a possible universal donor for marrow reconstitution and use in nuclear accidents. Life Sciences 2001; 69(13):1531-9.

24. Broxmeyer HE. Cord blood transplantation study standard operating procedures: An evolving document will improve cord blood unit quality (editorial). J Hematother 1998;7: 479-80.

25. Klingermann HG, Shepherd JD, Eaves CJ, Eaves AC. The role of erythropoietin and other growth factors in transfusion medicine. Transfus Med Rev 1991;5:33-47.

26. Goodnough LT, Anderson KC. Recombinant growth factors. Transfus Sci 1995;16:45-62.

27. Fischl M, Galpin JE, Levine JD, et al. Recombinant human erythropoietin for patients with AIDS treated with zidovudine. N Engl J Med 1990;322:1488-93.

28. Abels RI, Larholt KM, Krantz KD, et al. Recombinant human erythropoietin for the treatment of the anemia of cancer. In: Murphy MJ Jr, ed. Blood cell growth factors: Their present and future use in hematology and oncology. Dayton, OH: Alpha Med Press, 1991:121.

29. Demetri GD, Kris M, Wade J, et al. Quality-of-life benefit in chemotherapy patients treated with epoetin alpha is independent of disease response or tumor type: Results from a prospective community oncology study. J Clin Oncol 1998;16:3412-25.

30. Casadevall N, Nataf J, Viron B, et al. Pure red cell aplasia and antierythropoietin antibodies in patients treated with recombinant erythropoietin. N Engl J Med 2002:346; 469-75.

31. Nemunaitis J. Granulocyte-macrophage colony-stimulating factor: A review from preclinical development to clinical application. Transfusion 1993;33:70-83.

32. Bolwell BJ, Fishleder A, Anderson SW, et al. G-CSF primed peripheral blood progenitor cells in autologous marrow transplantation: Parameters affecting bone marrow engraftment. Bone Marrow Transplant 1993;12:609-14.

33. Dale DC, Liles WC, Llewellyn C, et al. Neutrophil transfusions: Kinetics and function of neutrophils mobilized with granulocyte-colony-stimulating factor and dexamethasone. Transfusion 1998;38:713-21.

34. Strauss RG. Neutrophil (granulocyte) transfusions in the new millennium. Transfusion 1998;38:710-12.

35. Nemunaitis J, Singer LW, Buckner CD. Use of recombinant human granulocyte-macrophage colony-stimulating factor in graft failure after bone marrow transplantation. Blood 1990;76:245-53.

36. American Society of Clinical Oncology. 1997 update of recommendations for the use of hematopoietic colony-stimulating factors: Evidence-based, clinical practice guidelines. J Clin Oncol 1997;15:3288.

37. Macdougall IC, Gray SJ, Elston O, et al. Pharmacokinetics of novel erythropoiesis stimulating protein compared with epoetin alfa in dialysis patients. J Am Soc Nephrol 1999;10:2392-5.

38. Locatelli F, Olivares J, Walker R, et al. Novel erythropoiesis stimulating protein for treatment of anemia in chronic renal insufficiency. Kidney Int 2001;60:741-7.

39. Lyman SD, Jacobsen SE. C-kit ligand and Flt3 ligand: Stem/progenitor cell factors with overlapping yet distinct activities. Blood 1998;91:1101-34.

40. Archimbaud E, Thomas X. Thrombopoietic factors potentially useful in the treatment of acute leukemia. Leuk Res 1998;22:1155-64.

41. Goodnough LT, Romo J, DiPersio J, et al. Thrombopoietin therapy increases platelet yields in healthy donors. Blood 2001;98:1339-45.

42. Kuter DJ. Thrombopoietin: Biology, clinical applications, role in the donor setting. J Clin Apheresis 1996;11:149-59.

43. Li J, Yang C, Xia Y, et al. Thrombocytopenia caused by the development of antibodies to thrombopoietin. Blood 2001;98:3241-8.

44. Sayers MH, Anderson KC, Goodnough LT, et al. Reducing the risk for transfusion-transmitted cytomegalovirus infection. Ann Intern Med 1992;116:55-62.

45. Friedberg RC. Transfusion therapy in the patient undergoing hematopoietic stem cell transplantation. Hematol Oncol Clin North Am 1994;8:1105-16.

46. Champlin RE, Horowitz MM, van Bekkum DW, et al. Graft failure following bone marrow transplanation for severe aplastic anemia: Risk factors and treatment results. Blood 1989;73:606-13.

47. Anderson KC. The role of the blood bank in hematopoietic stem cell transplantation. Transfusion 1992;32:272-85.

48. Petz LD. Immunohematologic problems associated with bone marrow transplanation. Transfus Med Rev 1987; 1:85-100.

49. Klumpp TR. Immunohematologic complications of bone marrow transplantation. Bone Marrow Transplant 1991;8 (3):159-70.

50. Anderlini P, Korbling M. The use of mobilized peripheral blood stem cells from normal donors for allografting. Stem Cells 1997;15:9-17.

51. Majolino I, Saglio G, Scime R, et al. High incidence of chronic GVHD after primary allogeneic peripheral blood stem cell transplantation in patients with hematologic malignancies. Bone Marrow Transplant 1996;17(4):555-60.

52. Paulin T, Ringden O, Lonnquist B, et al. The importance of pre-bone-marrow transplantation serology in determining subsequent cytomegalovirus infection. An analysis of risk factors. Scand J Infect Dis 1986;18:199-209.

53. Guidelines for preventing opportunistic infections among hematopoietic stem cell transplant recipients. Biol Blood Marrow Transplant 2000;6:659-713.

THERAPEUTIC APHERESIS

Description

Therapeutic apheresis involves the separation and removal of one or more abnormal constituents from a patient's blood in order to achieve a clinical benefit.[1] Specific procedures are defined by the blood component removed: cytapheresis (any cellular element), leukapheresis, lymphapheresis, erythrocytapheresis, platelet-pheresis, or plasmapheresis (plasma exchange). While several of these procedures can be performed manually, the use of automated cell separators permits processing of larger quantities of blood, more efficient component separation, and simultaneous reinfusion of remaining blood constituents.

Indications

Cytapheresis

Therapeutic cytapheresis can be used to reduce either quantitatively excessive or qualitatively abnormal cellular elements in the blood. This technique is commonly employed in emergency situations when conventional therapies are ineffective or slow to take effect. The clinical benefit is often acute and rapid, but temporary.

Erythrocytapheresis with red cell exchange has been used to manage acute severe complications of sickle cell disease (stroke, priapism, acute chest syndrome, retinal artery occlusion) and for long-term prophylaxis or prevention of recurrence of strokes, by decreasing the level of hemoglobin S to less than 30%.[2] Erythrocytapheresis is effective in managing iron overload associated with chronically transfused patients with sickle cell disease.[3] Other indications for erythrocytapheris are rare. It has been used to treat overwhelming parasitic infections with malaria and babesia[1] and immune hemolysis in the transplant setting.

Cytapheresis is also useful in the management of extreme leukocytosis and thrombocytosis in patients with acute leukemia or myeloproliferative disorders. Hyperleukocytic syndrome is characterized by central nervous system and/or pulmonary symptoms due to reduced blood flow associated with increased viscosity from excessive white cells in the microcirculation. By achieving immediate, although temporary, reductions in circulating white cells, leukapheresis can successfully treat life-threatening leukostasis in patients with blast counts >50,000 to 100,000/μL. Cell type appears to be important, with symptoms appearing more frequently in patients with acute myelogenous leukemia (particularly M4 or M5 types) than in patients with chronic lymphocytic leukemia or chronic myelogenous leukemia. Multiple procedures may be required in combination with cytotoxic therapy to maintain lower counts due to intravascular migration of tumor cells.

In patients with myeloproliferative disorders and severe symptomatic thrombocytosis, plateletpheresis can be useful in the prevention of thrombotic and hemorrhagic complications by acutely lowering the platelet count. Typically, plateletpheresis is initiated when the platelet count exceeds 1,000,000/μL. The platelet count is typically transiently lowered by 30% to 50% after a single procedure.[4]

Plasmapheresis

Therapeutic plasmapheresis has found widespread clinical application in autoimmune, hematologic, renal, metabolic, and neurologic disorders. The American Society for Apheresis has categorized the evidence for efficacy of plasmaphersis for various indications into four categories: standard therapy for the disease; evidence favors efficacy, but not first-line therapy; inadequate evidence for evaluation; and no demonstrated efficacy in controlled trials.[5] Table 7 shows the most common indications for plasmapheresis and the category of supportive evidence.[6,7] Most plasma

Table 7. Indications for Therapeutic Plasmapheresis

Indication	Category of Evidence
Neurologic Disorders	
Guillain-Barré syndrome	I
Myasthenia gravis	I
Eaton-Lambert syndrome	I
Chronic inflammatory demyelinating polyneuropathy	I
Amyotrophic lateral sclerosis	IV
Multiple sclerosis	III
Hematologic Disorders	
Thrombotic thrombocytopenic purpura	I
Hemolytic-uremic syndrome	II
Hyperviscosity syndrome	I
Cryoglobulinemia	I
Cold agglutinin disease	III
Idiopathic thrombocytopenic purpura	III (II with immuno-adsorption column)
Posttransfusion purpura	I
Coagulation factor inhibitors	III
Rheumatologic Disorders	
Rheumatoid arthritis	IV (II with immuno-adsorption column)
Systemic lupus erythematosus	II
Vasculitis	II
Polymyositis/dermatomyositis	IV
Scleroderma	III
Renal Diseases	
Goodpasture's syndrome	I
Rapidly progressive glomerulonephritis	II
Renal allograft rejection	IV
Metabolic Disorders	
Hypercholesterolemia	I (for selective adsorption)
Grave's disease/thyroid storm	III
Hepatic failure	III
Miscellaneous Disorders	
HIV-related peripheral neuropathy	I
Pemphigus	II
Psoriasis	IV
Drug/toxin removal	II
Heart, lung, liver rejection	III

(I) standard therapy for the disease, (II) evidence favors efficacy, but not first-line therapy, (III) inadequate evidence for evaluation, (IV) no demonstrated efficacy in controlled trials

Modified with permission from Kaplan AA. A practical guide to therapeutic plasma exchange. Malden, MA: Blackwell Science, 1999:86-8.

exchange regimens include the processing of 1 to 1.5 plasma volumes for each of six procedures, performed over a 10- to 14-day period. The large amounts of plasma removed necessitate concurrent replacement with colloid, crystalloid, or a combination of solutions. Patients with thrombotic thrombocytopenic purpura are treated daily with fresh frozen plasma (or donor retested plasma) as a replacement solution until there is normalization of the platelet count and cessation of hemolysis. Patients who do not respond to daily plasmapheresis with plasma may be treated with cryo-supernatant as the replacement solution.[1]

Staphylococcal Protein A Immunoadsorption

Protein A derived from *Staphylococcus aureus* can be complexed to a carrier such as silicon and can be used for the ex-vivo absorption of monomeric IgG (subclasses 1, 2, and 4) and immune-complexed IgG. The Staphylococcal Protein A column has been approved for use in the treatment of chronic immune thrombocytopenic purpura and medically refractory rheumatoid arthritis. It has also been used in chemotherapy-associated hemolytic-uremic syndrome. Side effects of the Staphyloccocal Protein A column are observed in approximately 20% to 30% of patients and include pain (musculoskeletal), nausea/vomiting, fever, chills, and rash. Hypotension has been observed in patients on angiotensin-converting enzyme (ACE) inhibitors due to contact activation of kininogens and generation of bradykinin. Patients should discontinue taking ACE inhibitors at least 24 hours prior to treament with a Staphyloccocal Protein A column. Rare reported complications include anaphylactoid reactions, vasculitis, and thrombosis.

Selective Lipid Removal (Lipopheresis)

Lipopheresis can be used to reduce low-density lipoprotein (LDL) and lipoprotein(a) in patients with familial hypercholesterolemia who are unresponsive to lipid lowering therapy. Lipopheresis consists of plasma separation followed by either adsorption of LDL onto negatively charged dextran sulfate or LDL-antibody-coated sepharose beads, or precipitation of LDL by negatively charged heparin. Procedures are usually performed every 2 weeks, and a single procedure will lower the LDL cholesterol by 70% to 80%.[8]

Photopheresis

A special hemapheresis technique called photopheresis has been found to be efficacious in selected malignant and autoimmune disorders. The technique involves the exposure of peripheral blood leukocytes to the ingested drug 8-methoxypsoralen. Psoralen binds to DNA in all nucleated cells and, upon stimulation with ultraviolet light, prevents DNA replication. Within hours of psoralen ingestion, patients undergo a leukapheresis procedure, during which time isolated leukocytes are exposed to ultraviolet A irradiation and then returned to the patient. Photopheresis has become standard therapy for advanced forms of cutaneous T-cell lymphoma and Sezary syndrome, and has shown promise in the management of other autoimmune diseases, solid organ transplant rejection, and graft-vs-host disease after allogeneic marrow transplantation.[1,9]

Procedural Considerations

Vascular access is an important clinical issue in apheresis patients. Antecubital veins are preferred but may be too small. Fistulas, grafts, or shunts are ready sites of vascular access. If central venous catheters are used for apheresis, then specialized non-collapsible types (eg, dialysis catheters) must be used. Saline or heparin must be used to maintain catheter patency. Chronic cannulation of the femoral vein is associated with an increased risk of catheter thombosis and should be avoided if possible. The replacement of fluid volume lost during these procedures can be accomplished using saline, 5% albumin, or a combination of the two. Due to the extracorporeal volume, patients weighing less than 10 to 20 kilograms may require red cells to prime the apheresis instrument. Plasma is rarely indicated due to the risk of transfusion-transmitted diseases. However, plasma is the required replacement solution in patients with thrombotic thrombocytopenic purpura and may be indicated for replenishing coagulation factors in other conditions if repeated daily procedures lead to a dilutional coagulopathy.

Complications of Therapeutic Apheresis

Complications associated with apheresis include sudden fluid shifts leading to hypotension, volume overload, or vasovagal reactions. Citrate-induced hypocalcemia may result in peri-oral tingling or numbness and paresthesias. Rarely, severe hypocalcemia may be associated with electrocardiogram abnormalities and dysrhythmias. Manifestations of hypocalcemia are more likely in large-volume procedures or procedures in which plasma is used as the replacement solution. Symptoms can usually be treated with oral calcium supplements. Intravenous calcium replacement (calcium gluconate or calcium chloride) may also be used.

Flushing and hypotension have been reported in patients taking ACE inhibitors receiving albumin replacement during standard apheresis.[10] ACE inhibitors block the degradation of bradykinins present in albumin solutions. It is recommended that patients discontinue taking ACE inhibitors at least 24 hours prior to an apheresis procedure.

Concentrations of some drugs, particularly those that are protein bound (eg, antibiotics, anticoagulants, sedatives), and immune globulin preparations may be lowered by plasmapheresis. Whenever possible, daily medications should be administered *after* plasmapheresis.

Rare reactions include catheter thrombosis and/or infection, air embolism, cardiac arrhythmias, seizures, anaphylaxis (with plasma infusions), and cardiorespiratory arrest. In patients undergoing repeated procedures, coagulation factors and plasma IgG levels may fall considerably. Depletion coagulopathy can be mitigated by partial plasma replacement at the end of the procedure. Severely immunosuppressed patients may benefit from immune globulin infusions when IgG levels are reduced to below 200 mg/dL.[1]

References

1. McLeod BC, Price TH, Drew MJ, eds. Apheresis: Principles and practice. Bethesda, MD: AABB Press, 1997.
2. Adams RJ, McKie VC, Hsu L, et al. Prevention of a first stroke by transfusions in children with sickle cell anemia and abnormal results on transcranial Doppler ultrasonography. N Engl J Med 1998;339(1):5-11.
3. Kim HC, Dugan NP, Silber JH, et al. Erythrocytapheresis therapy to reduce iron overload in chronically transfused patients with sickle cell disese. Blood 1994;83:1136-42.
4. Klein HG. Principles of apheresis: In: Anderson KC, Ness PM, eds. Scientific basis of transfusion medicine. Philadelphia, PA: WB Saunders, 2000:553-68.
5. McLeod BC. Clinical application of therapeutic apheresis. J Clin Apheresis 2000;15:1-5.
6. Kaplan AA. A practical guide to therapeutic plasma exchange. Malden, MA: Blackwell Science, 1999:85-8.
7. Leitman SF, Ciavarella D, McLeod B, et al. Guidelines for therapeutic hemapheresis. Bethesda, MD: American Association of Blood Banks, 1994.
8. Winters JL, Pineda AA, McLeod BC, et al. Therapeutic apheresis in renal and metabolic diseases. J Clin Apharsis 2000;15:53-73.
9. Strauss RG, Ciavarella D, Gilcher RO, et al. Clinical applications of therapeutic hemapheresis: An overview of current management. J Clin Apheresis 1993;8:189-94.
10. Owen HG, Brecher ME. Atypical reactions associated with use of angiotensin-converting enzyme inhibitors and apheresis. Transfusion 1994;34:891-4.

INDEX

T

Transplantation
  hematopoietic progenitor
    cells, 137-144
  solid organ, 78-79
Trypanosoma cruzi, 130
TT virus, 129
TTP. *See* Thrombotic
  thrombocytopenic purpura
Type and screens, 61-62

U

Uremia, 95
Urgent transfusions, 66-67

V

Variant Creutzfeldt-Jakob disease,
  130
Vascular access in apheresis, 161
Viruses
  in Factor VIII products, 40

  in Immune Globulin, 52
  pathogen inactivation, 30-31
  in plasma products, 25, 26
  transfusion-transmitted,
    127-129
Vitamin K deficiency, 99-100
Volume expanders, synthetic, 49-50
von Willebrand disease (vWD), 28,
  40, 90-91, 95-96

W

Warfarin, 100
Whole Blood
  characteristics in storage of, *7*
  composition and volume of, *2*
  contraindications and precau-
    tions for, 8
  description of, 6
  dose and administration of, 8
  indications for, *2*, 6, 8
  use in massive transfusions,
    68